Carnegie Commission on the Future of Higher Education.

Higher Education and the Nation's Health

POLICIES FOR MEDICAL AND DENTAL EDUCATION

A Special Report and Recommendations by
The Carnegie Commission on Higher Education

OCTOBER 1970

MCGRAW-HILL BOOK COMPANY

New York   St. Louis   San Francisco   Düsseldorf
London   Sydney   Toronto   Mexico   Panama
Rio de Janeiro   Singapore

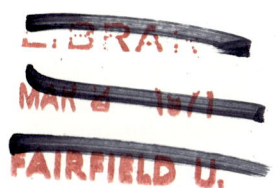

The views and conclusions expressed in this report are solely those of the members of the Carnegie Commission on Higher Education and do not necessarily reflect the views or opinions of the Carnegie Corporation of New York, The Carnegie Foundation for the Advancement of Teaching, or their trustees, officers, directors, or employees.

Copyright © 1970 by The Carnegie Foundation for the Advancement of Teaching. All rights reserved. Printed in the United States of America.

Additional copies of this report may be ordered from McGraw-Hill Book Company, Hightstown, New Jersey 08520. The price is $2.95 a copy.

"The health of all the people is really the foundation upon which all their happiness and all their powers as a state depend."

BENJAMIN DISRAELI

Foreword

The Carnegie Commission on Higher Education will issue its final report and recommendations in 1972, after all its research projects have been completed. But many problems in higher education are urgent and need early action. The Commission submits special reports on such matters as soon as it has had an opportunity to review the relevant issues and develop specific recommendations.

This present report, *Higher Education and the Nation's Health: Policies for Medical and Dental Education,* is concerned with the serious shortage of professional health manpower, the need for expanding and restructuring the education of professional health personnel, and the vital importance of adapting the education of health manpower to the changes needed for an effective system of delivery of health care in the United States.

To the many persons who were consulted and gave us helpful suggestions, we wish to express our appreciation. Particularly valuable contributions were made by Dr. Mark S. Blumberg, former director of health planning, University of California, and Dr. Robert Tschirgi, professor of neurosciences, School of Medicine, University of California, San Diego.

The Commission is also especially indebted to the members of its Advisory Committee on Medical Education, which includes—in addition to Dr. Blumberg and Dr. Tschirgi—Dr. Julius H. Comroe, director, Cardiovascular Research Institute, University of California, San Francisco; Dr. Robert Glaser, vice-president for medical affairs and dean, School of Medicine, Stanford University; Dr. Clifford Grobstein, vice-chancellor for health sciences and dean, School of Medicine, University of California, San Diego; Dr. David A. Hamburg, executive head, Department of Psychiatry, School of Medicine, Stanford University; Dr. Phillip R. Lee, chancellor, University of California, San Francisco; and Dr. James A. Shannon, professor and special assistant to the president, The Rockefeller University.

We also appreciate the contributions of participants in conferences held in New York City on January 29, 1969, and June 8, 1970, including Dr. Robert S. Anderson, director, Comprehensive Health Services Program, Meharry Medical College; Dr. William Anlyan, vice-president for health affairs, Duke University Medical Center; Dr. Allan M. Cartter, chancellor, New York University; Dr. John Cooper, president, Association of American Medical Colleges; Dr. John T. Dunlop, David A. Wells professor of political economy, Harvard University; Dr. Robert Ebert, dean, Harvard Medical School; Dr. Rashi Fein, Center for Community Health and Medical Care, Harvard Medical School; Dr. Jon Joyce, Office of the Assistant Secretary for Planning and Evaluation, Department of Health, Education, and Welfare; Dr. Terrance Keenan, Commonwealth Fund of New York; Dr. Charles V. Kidd, director, Council on Federal Relations, Association of American Universities; Dr. Roy Lindahl, dental project director, Health Services Research Department, School of Dentistry, University of North Carolina; Margaret Mahoney, associate secretary and executive associate, Carnegie Corporation of New York; Dr. William Mayer, dean, School of Medicine, University of Missouri; Dr. Walsh McDermott, chairman, Department of Public Health, Cornell University Medical Center; Joseph Murtaugh, Association of American Medical Colleges; Dr. Quigg Newton, president, Commonwealth Fund of New York; Dr. Malcolm Peterson, director, Health Services Research and Development Center, Johns Hopkins University School of Medicine; Dr. Frederick C. Robbins, dean, School of Medicine, Case Western Reserve University; Dr. Ronald T. Taylor, Harvard Dental School; Dr. James V. Warren, chairman, Department of Medicine, Ohio State University College of Medicine; and Dr. John M. Weir, director, medical and natural sciences, The Rockefeller Foundation.

The Commission also received useful and constructive comments from Dr. Robert Graham, chairman, Joint Commission on Medical Education, Student American Medical Association; Dr. Seymour E. Harris, professor of economics and medical economics, University of California, San Diego; Dr. John S. Millis, vice-president, National Fund for Medical Education; Dr. David E. Rogers, vice-president for medical affairs and dean, School of Medicine, Johns Hopkins University, as well as several other members of the Hopkins medical faculty; Dr. C. H. William Ruhe, director, and Dr. Hayden Nicholson, Division of Medical Education, American Medical Association; Dr. Paul J. Sanazaro, director, National Center for Health Services Research and Development, U.S. Public Health Service; and a number of others, including medical students.

Particularly valuable reference sources in the preparation of the report were a study of the financing of medical education by Dr. Rashi Fein and Dr. Gerald Weber, soon to be published by McGraw-Hill for the Carnegie Commission, and a report on a seminar on medical education conducted at Harvard University in 1969 by Dr. John T. Dunlop and Dr. Robert Ebert.

We also wish to thank the members of our staff, and especially Dr. Margaret S. Gordon, for their work in preparing this report.

Eric Ashby
The Master
Clare College
Cambridge, England

Ralph M. Besse
Chairman of the Board
The Cleveland Electric Illuminating
  Company

Joseph P. Cosand
President
The Junior College District
  of St. Louis

William Friday
President
University of North Carolina

The Honorable Patricia
  Roberts Harris
Partner
Strasser, Spiegelberg, Fried, Frank,
  and Kampelman, Attorneys
Washington, D.C.

David D. Henry
President
University of Illinois

Theodore M. Hesburgh,
  C.S.C.
President
University of Notre Dame

Stanley J. Heywood
President
Eastern Montana College

Carl Kaysen
Director
Institute for Advanced Study
  at Princeton

Kenneth Keniston
Professor of Psychology
School of Medicine, Yale University

Katharine E. McBride
President
Bryn Mawr College

James A. Perkins
Chairman and Director
Center for Educational Enquiry

Clifton W. Phalen
Chairman of the Executive
  Committee
Marine Midland Banks, Inc.

Nathan M. Pusey
President
Harvard University

David Riesman
Professor of Social Sciences
Harvard University

The Honorable William W. Scranton

Norton Simon

Kenneth Tollett
Professor of Law
Texas Southern University

Clark Kerr
Chairman

Contents

Foreword, v

1 *Major Themes,* 1

2 *The Crisis in Health Care Delivery and Health Manpower,* 13
The problem of unmet need ▪ The problem of rising expectations ▪ The problem of insufficient health manpower ▪ The problem of ineffective financing ▪ The problem of rising costs ▪ Summary

3 *The Scope of This Report,* 23

4 *Medical Education Today,* 25
The 60 years since Flexner ▪ Doctors, dentists, and their assistants

5 *The Future of Health Care Delivery,* 31

6 *The Future of Health Manpower Education,* 35
The evidence of a shortage of physicians and dentists ▪ The expansion of health manpower education ▪ The role of university health science centers ▪ Acceleration of medical and dental education ▪ Integration of the curriculum ▪ Other curriculum reforms ▪ The location of new university health science centers ▪ The role of area health education centers ▪ The location of area health education centers

7 *Financial Support and the Federal Government,* 61
Student grants ▪ Student loans ▪ A national health service corps ▪ Tuition policy ▪ Cost-of-instruction supplements to institutions ▪ Construction grants and loans ▪ Start-up grants ▪ Support of research ▪ National and regional planning ▪ Recertification ▪ Studies of health manpower ▪ A national health manpower commission ▪ Estimated cost of recommended federal aid

8 *The Role of the States,* 81

9 *The Role of the Universities,* 91

10 *The Role of the Comprehensive Colleges and Community Colleges,* 95

11 *The Role of the Foundations,* 97

12 *Carnegie Commission Goals To Be Achieved by 1980,* 99

Appendix A: Joint Statements of the American Medical Association and the Association of American Medical Colleges, March 5, 1968, and April 16, 1968, 101

Appendix B: Tables, 107

References, 125

Higher Education and the Nation's Health

1. Major Themes

1 *"Life . . . and the pursuit of happiness"* Americans deserve and can afford better health care. We have the highest standard of living, but not the highest standard of life—as measured by infant mortality and average life expectancy. A number of countries surpass us. In fact, in comparison with other nations, we are losing. Better health care is clearly a high national priority.

2 *The four components of better health care* To improve health care requires:

- More and better health manpower
- More and better health care facilities
- Better financing arrangements for the health care of the population
- Better planning for health manpower and health care delivery

This report is concerned with more and better health manpower, particularly at the level of doctors and dentists. The Commission believes that the provision of highly skilled health manpower is a special responsibility of higher education. The adequacy of health care facilities, however, is the responsibility, not of universities and colleges, but of federal, state, and local health authorities. As to the financing of individual care, the report assumes that as the result of public and private efforts, some form of health insurance will be available to all American citizens within this decade. Planning is partly a responsibility of higher education, particularly the planning for health personnel, but mostly of public agencies.

All four components of better health care mentioned above must be carefully developed in order to yield maximum benefits. This report is primarily concerned with only one major aspect of these components—the contributions of university health science centers. Most health care personnel are trained outside these centers, and we recommend that the total spectrum of health care personnel be reviewed by a National Health Manpower Commission.

3 *A serious manpower shortage* The United States today faces only one serious manpower shortage, and that is in health care personnel. This shortage can become even more acute as health insurance expands, leading to even more unmet needs and greater cost inflation, unless corrective action is taken now. It takes a long lead time to get more doctors and dentists.

4 *Higher education and health* Higher education, as it trains the most skilled health personnel, has a great responsibility for the welfare of the nation. What colleges of agriculture once did for a rural society can now be done for an urban society by the health science centers—and that is to improve the quality of life for nearly all people in their areas.

The Carnegie Commission is giving special attention to medical and dental education because of their high importance to national welfare, their greatly increased complexity, and their heavy burden of costs. We have elsewhere identified the greatest priorities for higher education in the 1970s as being: (1) to provide greater equality of educational opportunity for all our youth, (2) to undertake reform and innovation, and (3) to provide more health care personnel. All three of these priorities are involved in this report. We know of no single area in all of higher education where more constructive action can be taken now than in medical and dental education.

5 *A propitious time to act* This is a most favorable period for new and improved endeavors:
- The public has a great concern for health care.
- Existing medical and dental schools are expanding, and new ones are being built; and a period of growth can also be a period of change and improvement.
- The students of today are highly motivated to encourage and support constructive change.

- The medical and dental schools have a number of remarkably able leaders.
- The professional associations are open to new ideas and are anxious to find better ways to provide better health care—to their great credit and to the nation's great advantage.

As a consequence, medical and dental education are undergoing more constructive self-examination than they have since the Flexner report of 1910—and more self-examination is going on than in any other field of higher education. The second great transformation of medical education and research is now underway, and the United States, once again, will greatly benefit.

6 *The goals* We see these as major objectives:

- To provide more health care personnel of the right kinds
- To achieve a better geographic distribution of personnel and educational facilities, particularly for the sake of the central city and rural areas
- To ensure more equality of opportunity for women and members of minority groups
- To provide more appropriate training for the work actually to be performed and, in doing so, to respond to the constructive suggestions of students
- To relate health care education more effectively to health care delivery
- To bring about a more equitable distribution of the financial burden between the federal government and the states, and among the several states
- To limit costs to the greatest extent possible

We shall make recommendations toward achieving each of these goals. To the extent that they are achieved, inflation will be slowed and, at the same time, health care will be improved.

7 *The Flexner model and new models* The Flexner model, based on Johns Hopkins, Harvard, and, before them, German medical education, called for emphasis on biological research. Science was to be at the base of medical education. The Flexner model has been the sole fully accepted model in the United States since 1910. Some schools have fulfilled its promise brilliantly; others have been pale imitations; but all have tried to follow it. It has led to great strides forward in the quality of research and the quality of individual medical practitioners. The Flexner, or *research* model, however, looked inward to science in the medical school itself. It is a self-contained approach. Consequently, it has two weaknesses in modern times: (1) it largely ignores health care delivery outside the medical school and its own hospital, and (2) it sets science in the medical school apart from science on the general campus with resulting duplication of effort. This second weakness is now being highlighted by the extension of medical concerns beyond science into economics, sociology, engineering, and many other fields. Medical schools have had their own departments of biochemistry, but to add their own departments of economics and sociology and engineering would accentuate the problem of duplication of faculty and equipment. Also, the better economists would rather be in a department of economics on a general campus than separated from their colleagues in a department of medical economics: members of other disciplines would have similar preferences. The self-contained Flexner model thus leads to expensive duplication and can lead to some loss in quality.

Two new models are arising: (1) the *health care delivery* model, where the medical school, in addition to training, does research in health care delivery, advises local hospitals and health authorities, works with community colleges and comprehensive colleges on the training of allied health personnel, carries on continuing education for health personnel, and generally orients itself to external service; and (2) the *integrated science* model, where most or all of the basic science (and social science) instruction is carried on within the main campus (or other general campuses) and not duplicated in the medical school, which provides mainly clinical instruction. In this model (as in England), the medical school may be, essentially, a teaching hospital; but this is not necessary—it may, rather, carry on all its "Flexner" functions except the traditional first one or two years of science education.

Mixtures are of course possible and are occurring among these "pure" types. The research and health care delivery models may be combined, as is being done at Harvard and Johns Hopkins; the research and integrated science models may be combined, as is being proposed at Michigan and for the new Harvard–MIT endeavor; and the health care delivery and integrated science models may be combined, as at the new medical schools of the University of Illinois. All three, of course, could also be combined.

We believe that the new interests in health care delivery and in the integration of science and other disciplinary efforts are wise. The simple Flexner research model is no longer adequate as the sole model. A few schools, and many parts of schools, will, and should, stay with the Flexner model, but we believe that the nation will be better served as many schools move in different directions. A diversity of models and mixtures of models is now desirable. Not only can the developing and new schools experiment; but as existing schools expand, they can direct their expansion in new directions so that there can be diversity *within* schools—for example, the next group of 40 additional students admitted might be asked to take their science on the main campus of the parent university. The "cluster-college" approach of changing and diversifying—rather than just duplicating on a larger scale—when expanding a general campus can be undertaken also in a health science center.

Pacesetter schools, such as those noted above, are moving toward health care delivery, or the integration of science, or both. We support these directions of movement. The nation has a sufficiency of the pure research model type of school. New developments should be toward greater integration with social needs, or toward greater integration with the general campus, or both.

8 *More doctors and dentists* We see a need for expanding the number of places for training doctors during this next decade by 50 percent, and of dentists by 20 percent. Many of these new places should be filled by women and members of minority groups.

9 *More allied health personnel* The current ratio of all health care personnel to doctors is about 10 to 1; in the long run we see this ratio rising substantially. We particularly favor expanded training of medical associates who can work under the general supervision of doctors and expanded training of medical assistants who can work under the doctors' specific directions. We regard as especially promising the Medex program of training medical corpsmen with military experience to become doctor's assistants, and we note that as many as 3,000 a year might be trained with an all-out effort. We believe such an all-out effort is unlikely, however, and we estimate

that by the end of this decade about 3,500 associates and assistants may be trained each year. The public, of course, will need to be willing to accept the services of these associates and assistants, as they do in some other countries, and we believe they will. We similarly suggest the training of dental associates and dental assistants. Colorado, Duke, and Washington are among the universities now giving leadership in these directions.

Most of the allied health personnel will be trained in comprehensive colleges and community colleges, and their roles in this area will greatly expand. Allied health personnel can be trained more quickly and less expensively than doctors and dentists, and their availability will make possible the better use of the time and skill of doctors and dentists. Primary emphasis should be placed on increasing the supply of allied health personnel.

10 *To serve all the people everywhere* We believe in the geographic dispersion of health training centers, as our recommendations will make clear. The Flexner model school could be located anywhere, for research results are easily transported. The *health care delivery* model needs to be located where the people live.

11 *New health science centers* Twenty-seven health science centers are now being started around the United States. It is said that seventy more are being considered. We see a need for nine more (see Map 1) to give adequate regional coverage.

12 *Area health education centers* We recommend 126 area health education centers to serve localities without a health science center (see Map 2). Each of these centers would be at a local hospital. The centers' educational programs would be administered by university health science centers. They would train medical residents and M.D. and D.D.S. candidates on a rotational basis; they would carry on continuing education for local doctors, dentists, and other health care personnel; they would advise with local health authorities and hospitals; they would assist community colleges and comprehensive colleges in training allied health personnel; and, in other ways, they would help improve health care in their areas. We consider this development of basic importance. It would put most of the local advantages of a health science center into many localities which do not warrant a full-scale center. This proposal would put

MAP 1 University health science centers and Carnegie Commission goals for new university health science centers by 1980, by state

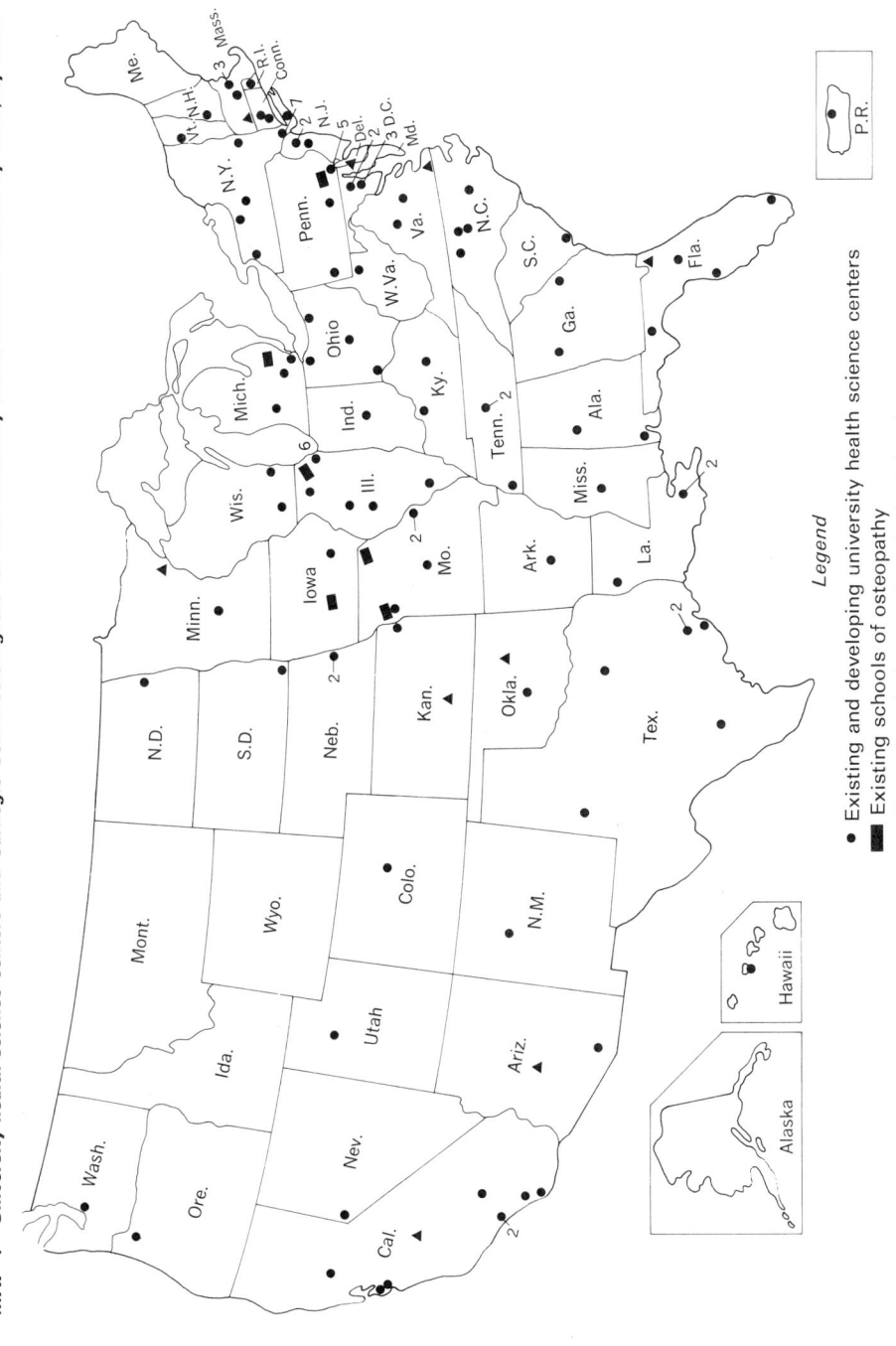

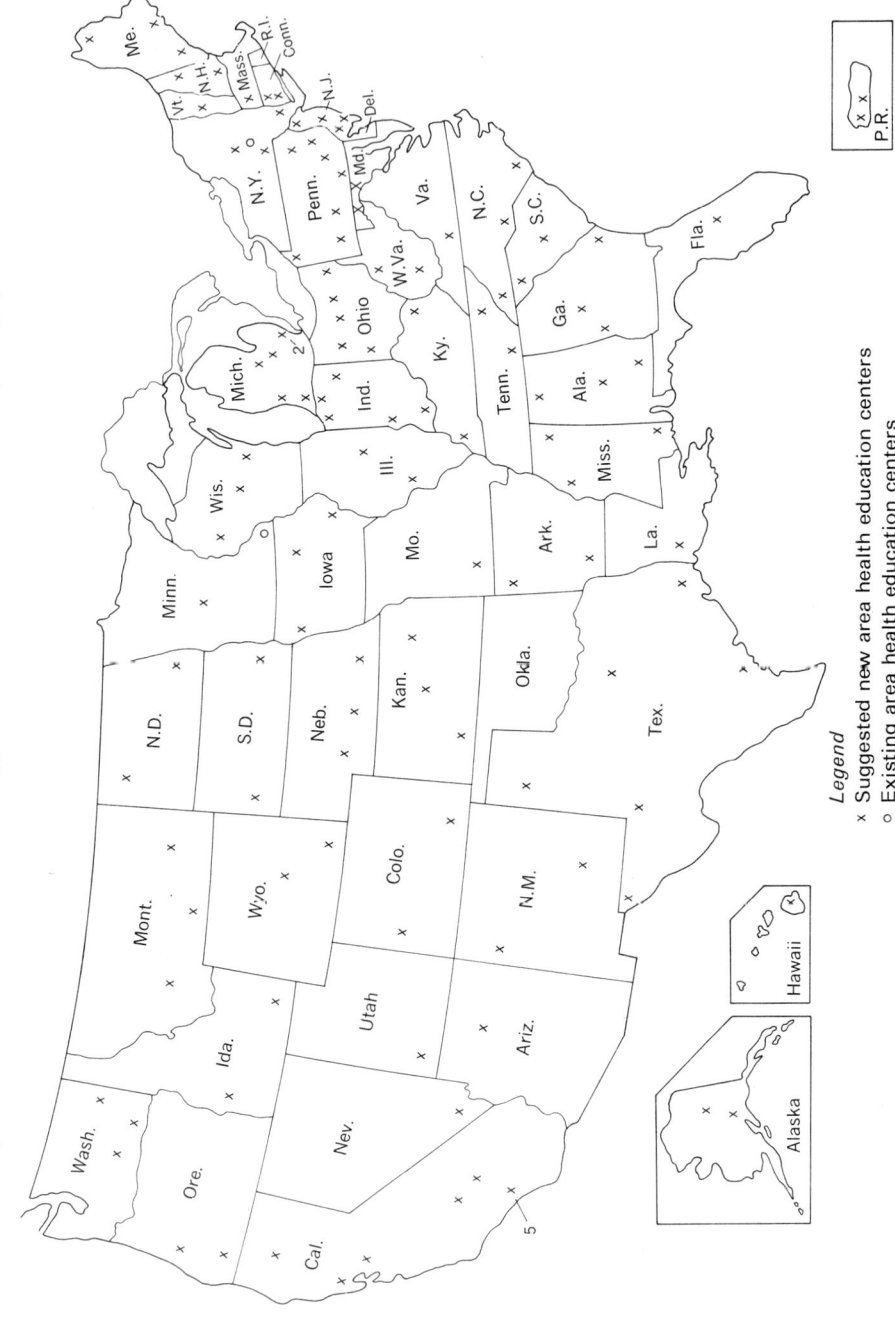

MAP 2 *Existing area health education centers and suggested area health education centers by 1980, by state*

essential health services within one hour of driving time for over 95 percent of all Americans and within this same amount of time for all health care personnel. Much of the nation would be served by a higher level of expertise than is now locally available.

13 *Reforms* We favor:

- Shortening the time it takes to become a practicing medical doctor from eight years after the B.A. to six years.

- Providing an extra mobility point or decision-making point for both the student and the school by creating a degree between the A.B. and the M.D. It would normally be awarded after students satisfy the general science requirements. It might be called a Master of Philosophy in Human Biology, or a Bachelor of Medicine, or a Master of Science in Human Biology. The student could decide at that point whether to go on to the M.D., move in the direction of the Ph.D., or take employment as a teacher or a medical assistant or associate (perhaps after some additional practical training). At this point, the school would also be in a good position to advise the prospective M.D. candidate and to judge his quality.

- Improving the curriculum by tying more closely together basic science and clinical instruction—they now too often stand as unrelated worlds. Improvement could also be achieved by tying clinical instruction to work with "garden-variety" as well as "exotic" patients; by creating several paths, rather than only one, for students depending on their prior background and their special interests—for example, a psychiatrist needs less basic science than a person intending to become a research scientist; and by having the students help determine the curriculum. Case Western Reserve recently has given notable leadership in curricular innovation.

- Improving the residency by giving the young doctor a wider variety of experience and more of it under skilled supervision.

- Creating a National Health Service Corps.

- Providing an Educational Opportunity Bank for medical and dental students.

- Improving the planning of health manpower.

14 *Sharing the financial burdens* We recommend:

- That the federal government meet more of the costs of medical and dental education. It already supports most of the costs of medical research. Doctors can and do move from state to state, and some states are reluctant to educate M.D's for practice elsewhere.
- That the states support private medical and dental schools.
- That the levels of support among states be more nearly equalized. Some states exploit the investment other states make in medical education.
- That both the federal government and the states seek reforms and improvements as they expend their funds.

15 *Cutting costs* The expanded health manpower and external service programs we recommend will cost substantial sums of money, but total expenditures should be held to the lowest reasonable levels. Costs could be reduced by:

- Reducing from four to three the years it takes to get an M.D. degree. This change alone, if adopted by all medical schools, would increase the number of student places available by one-third, without further construction costs and with little further operating costs. It would also result in student support savings and will get students into practice sooner. Dartmouth is developing a program designed to meet some of these objectives.
- Reducing from four to three the years it takes to fulfill residency requirements. This, too, will save costs and get doctors into practice earlier.
- Combining science work on the campus and in the medical school, thus reducing duplication.
- Reducing the ratio of faculty to students, which is particularly high in medical education.
- Entering two classes a year and thus making better use of laboratory facilities and teaching personnel.
- Teaching during the summer period.
- Holding federal research expenditures steady as a percentage of GNP after a period of spectacular rise.

- Greatly increasing the number of allied health personnel and thus raising the productivity of doctors and dentists.
- Raising the minimum size of a medical class to 100 and thus obtaining economies of scale.
- Using outside hospitals for clinical training rather than, or in addition to, subsidizing a "university hospital."

Expenditures of medical schools have gone up twice as fast in the past decade as expenditures in higher education generally, yet the number of students in medical schools has risen only half as fast as in the rest of higher education. It is high time to look more carefully at costs.

16 The nation has a good opportunity to improve the health care of its citizens. By its contribution to that improvement, higher education has a great opportunity to become more useful to society.

2. The Crisis in Health Care Delivery and Health Manpower

As the nation faces the 1970s, shortcomings in the system of delivery of health care in the world's most affluent society must have high priority among the issues calling for attention and decisive action. Shortages of health manpower play an important role in these deficiencies and they are likely to continue throughout the 1970s and probably into the 1980s.

The most serious shortages of professional personnel in any major occupation group in the United States are in the health services. Thus, one of the greatest challenges to higher education in the 1970s is to mobilize its resources to meet the need for expanding the education of professional health manpower. To accomplish this task the nation's medical and dental schools, along with educational institutions training allied health personnel, will need greatly augmented public financial support, but they will also need to give sustained attention to restructuring their educational and service programs to meet the nation's need for a more adequate system of delivery of health care.

THE PROBLEM OF UNMET NEED

The record of the United States in prolonging life expectancy and preventing infant mortality is not impressive when compared with the experience of many other industrial countries. Although the best medical care in this country is as good as any in the world, many Americans receive inferior care, and some health care needs go entirely untreated.

While life expectancy of both white and nonwhite males and females in the United States has gradually increased during the last half-century, the lengthening of life expectancy has leveled off during the last two decades. Among 22 industrial countries, the

TABLE 1 Expectation of life at birth in 22 industrial countries

	Males			Females	
Country	Years of life	Date	Country	Years of life	Date
Sweden	71.6	1961–1965	Netherlands	76.1	1966
Netherlands	71.1	1966	Norway	76.0	1961–1965
Norway	71.0	1961–1965	Sweden	75.7	1961–1965
Israel*	70.4	1967	France	75.4	1966
Denmark	70.1	1965–1966	Denmark	74.7	1965–1966
Switzerland	68.7	1958–1963	United States	74.2	1967
East Germany	68.5	1963–1966	Australia	74.2	1960–1962
New Zealand†	68.4	1960–1962	Canada	74.2	1960–1962
Canada	68.4	1960–1962	United Kingdom	74.2	1963–1965
Japan	68.4	1966	Switzerland	74.1	1958–1963
France	68.2	1966	New Zealand†	73.8	1960–1962
Ireland	68.1	1960–1962	Czechoslovakia	73.6	1966
United Kingdom	68.1	1963–1965	Israel*	73.6	1967
Australia	67.9	1960–1962	Japan	73.6	1966
Belgium	67.7	1959–1963	Belgium	73.5	1959–1963
West Germany	67.6	1964–1966	East Germany	73.5	1963–1966
Czechoslovakia	67.3	1966	West Germany	73.5	1964–1966
Italy	67.2	1960–1962	Austria	73.4	1967
United States	67.0	1967	Finland	72.6	1961–1965
Austria	66.6	1967	Italy	72.3	1960–1962
Finland	65.4	1961–1965	Ireland	71.9	1960–1962
Argentina	63.7	1960–1965	Argentina	69.5	1960–1965

*Jewish population only.
† European population.
SOURCE: United Nations, *Demographic Yearbook, 1968*, New York, 1969.

United States ranked nineteenth in male life expectancy and sixth in female life expectancy in 1967 (Table 1).[1]

If we consider infant mortality, we find a somewhat similar pattern, although there has been an encouraging acceleration of the decline in our infant mortality rate in the last few years and a slight

---

[1] If data for all countries for which they are available are included, from 1959 to 1966, the life expectancy of males in the United States dropped from thirteenth to twenty-second place and female life expectancy from seventh to tenth place (1, pp. 14–15). However, data for some of the underdeveloped countries are not very reliable.

improvement in our international ranking. However, our ranking in 1968 was still below that of 1960 (Chart 1). Contrary to a widely held impression, the fact that the United States infant mortality rate is below that of a number of other industrial countries is not entirely attributable to higher rates for nonwhite people. The rate of 19.7 infant deaths per 1,000 live births for white people in the United States in 1967 was above the overall rate for 10 other countries in that year (2, p. 57, and 3).[2]

Not only are our rankings low, but the gaps between the United States rates and those in the highest ranking industrial countries are substantial. Among the factors that perhaps explain this situation are our relatively heterogeneous population, the fact that some of the other industrial countries have placed greater emphasis on preventive care and mass education relating to healthful practices, and the fact that every other industrial country has either a national health insurance system or a national health service (4).

The evidence of unmet need for dental care is equally disturbing. In the period 1960 to 1962 it was found that about 20 percent of persons aged 45 to 54 in the United States had lost all their teeth and that this proportion rose sharply with advancing age (5). The National Health Survey of 1963–1964 indicated that nearly three-fifths of the population had not seen a dentist in the preceding year and that one-sixth of the population had never seen a dentist (6, p. 14).

THE PROBLEM OF RISING EXPECTATIONS *Increasingly, health care is coming to be regarded not only as a necessity but also as a right to which all persons are entitled.* The trend toward ensuring the right to health care is virtually certain to continue until all Americans are guaranteed access to adequate care without regard to means. In June 1970, the House of Delegates of the American Medical Association adopted the following statement:

> That the AMA reaffirm, as a statement of the primary purpose and responsibility of the Association and the medical profession, "the promotion of the art and science of medicine and the betterment of public health," and, as part of this purpose, apply all possible efforts to make medical services of high quality available to all individuals.

Increasingly experts predict that the United States will adopt a national health insurance system, perhaps within this decade.

---

[2] See *References* for complete citations.

Higher education and the nation's health 16

CHART 1 Infant mortality rates for 22 industrial countries,* 1960 and 1968†

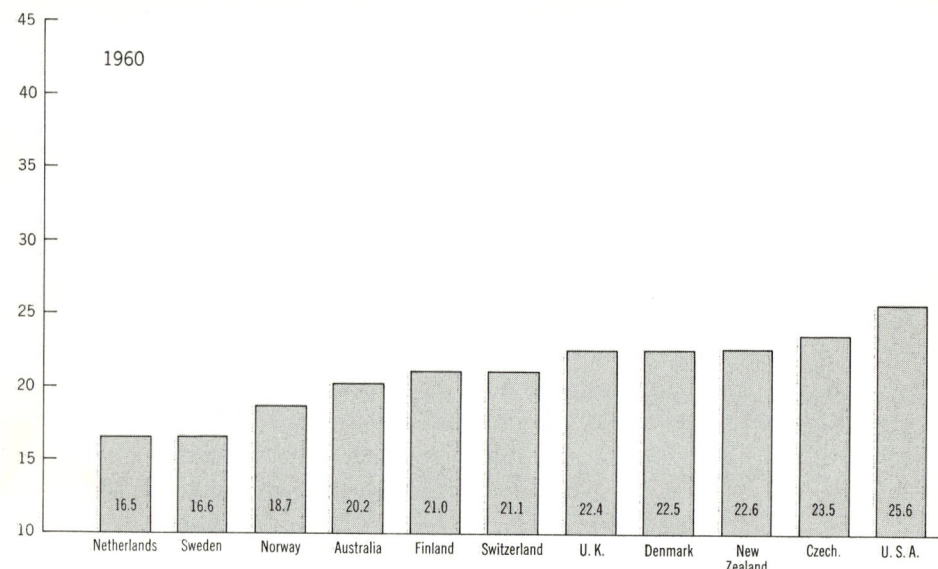

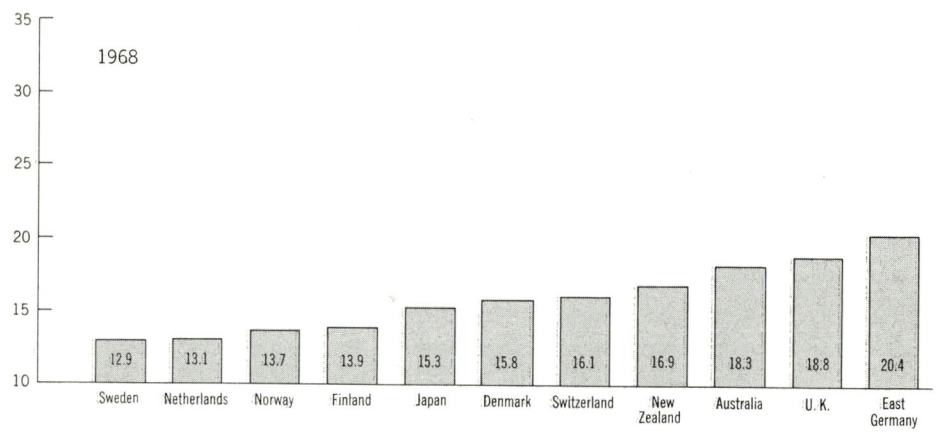

*Deaths under one year of age per 1,000 infants born alive.
† Data for Sweden, Australia, and Belgium are for 1967, and data for the Netherlands, Finland, Japan, and New Zealand are for 1969.
SOURCE: United Nations, Statistical Papers, *Population and Vital Statistics Report,* ser. A, vol. 14, no. 1, and vol. 22, no. 2.

The crisis in health care delivery and health manpower 17

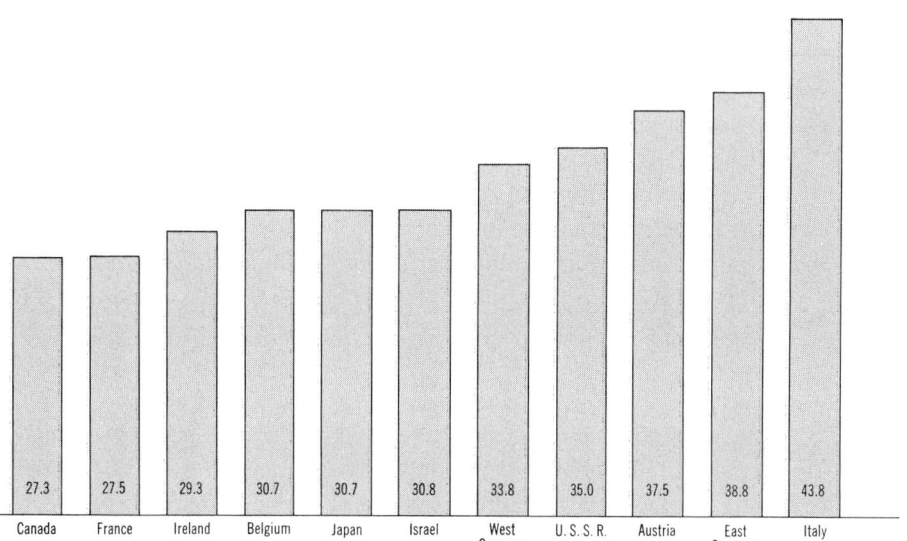

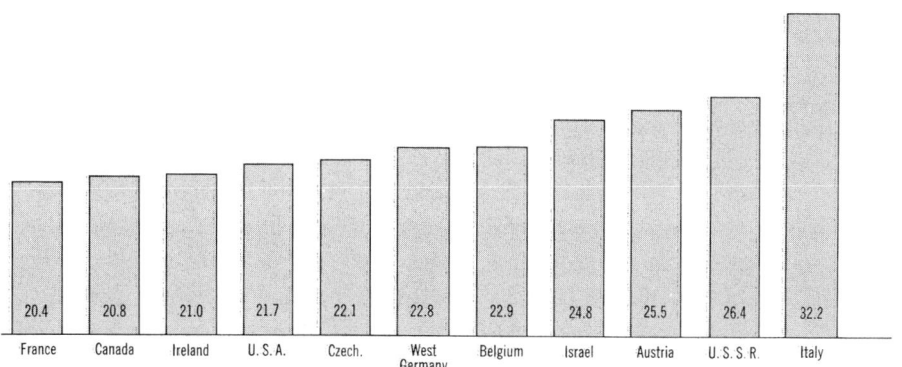

We accept this prediction. But, with the advent of national health insurance, the shortcomings in our methods of health care delivery and the critical shortages of our health manpower and facilities will become even more glaringly apparent. Unless we overcome these deficiencies, the present crisis in health care will appear to be a mere ripple in comparison with the mounting waves of problems to be faced when financial barriers to health care are lowered.

The recent proposal of the administration for a federal health insurance program for low- to moderate-income families with children (7), as a partial replacement for the Medicaid program, is an important step forward, but it will not go far toward meeting the need for a comprehensive national health insurance program. If only the elderly, now covered by Medicare, and relatively low-income persons are included in federal health insurance programs, the programs' costs per person will continue to be excessively high because these are high-cost, high-risk groups. The great advantage of a comprehensive national insurance system would be the inclusion of all the good risks along with the poor risks, resulting in much lower average costs.

THE PROBLEM OF INSUFFICIENT HEALTH MANPOWER

Although there is debate over the extent of shortages of health manpower, critical shortages do exist. Dr. Roger Egeberg, Assistant Secretary of the U.S. Department of Health, Education, and Welfare, recently stated that today the United States needs about 50,000 more physicians, "a couple of hundred thousand more nurses," and "almost 150,000 more technicians" (8, p. 73).

The geographic distribution of health manpower is highly uneven, and although there is no clear agreement on what ratio of, say, physicians to population is adequate, there is little question that the supply of health manpower is gravely deficient in some parts of the nation (Chart 2). Moreover, the fact that New York and Massachusetts have high ratios of physicians to population does not mean that a resident of a lower-income neighborhood of New York City or Boston has adequate access to a physician. As one writer on our "ailing medical system" recently put it (9, p. 86):

Private physicians are as hard to find in some neighborhoods of New York City as in backward rural counties of the South.

The uneven geographic distribution of health manpower is, of course, related to differences in per capita income among states and local areas and resulting differences in family expenditures on

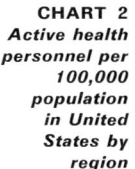

CHART 2
Active health personnel per 100,000 population in United States by region

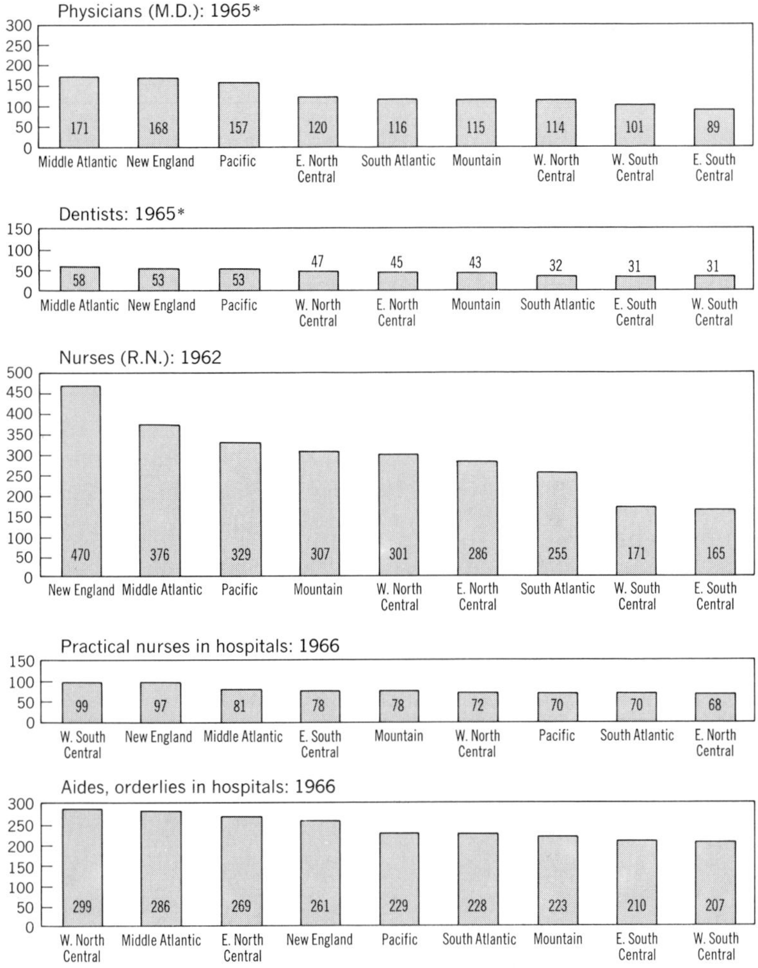

Physicians (M.D.): 1965*

Middle Atlantic	New England	Pacific	E. North Central	South Atlantic	Mountain	W. North Central	W. South Central	E. South Central
171	168	157	120	116	115	114	101	89

Dentists: 1965*

Middle Atlantic	New England	Pacific	W. North Central	E. North Central	Mountain	South Atlantic	E. South Central	W. South Central
58	53	53	47	45	43	32	31	31

Nurses (R.N.): 1962

New England	Middle Atlantic	Pacific	Mountain	W. North Central	E. North Central	South Atlantic	W. South Central	E. South Central
470	376	329	307	301	286	255	171	165

Practical nurses in hospitals: 1966

W. South Central	New England	Middle Atlantic	E. South Central	Mountain	W. North Central	Pacific	South Atlantic	E. North Central
99	97	81	78	78	72	70	70	68

Aides, orderlies in hospitals: 1966

W. North Central	Middle Atlantic	E. North Central	New England	Pacific	South Atlantic	Mountain	E. South Central	W. South Central
299	286	269	261	229	228	223	210	207

*Nonfederal per 100,000 civilian population.
SOURCE: U.S. Public Health Service, *Health Manpower, Perspective: 1967*, Washington, D.C., 1967, p. 14.

health care. But these variations are also related to differences in education, in the size of communities in which people live, and to racial background (10). Merely increasing the supply of physicians will not solve the problem of deficient health care in low-income areas. As we move toward a more adequate system of financing medical care, we may also need to devise special financial and nonfinancial incentives to induce physicians and other health personnel to work in low-income areas.

We also need to intensify our efforts to overcome inefficiencies in the use of health personnel. Expensively trained physicians are performing tasks that could well be carried out by less broadly trained personnel. Hospital personnel are also wastefully used in all too many instances. In fact, some critics of our health care delivery system go so far as to call it a "nonsystem." As the National Advisory Commission on Health Manpower put it (11, vol. 1, p. 3):

> Medical care in the U.S. is more a collection of bits and pieces with overlapping duplication, great gaps, high costs and wasted effort than an integrated system in which needs and efforts are closely related.

THE PROBLEM OF INEFFECTIVE FINANCING

Americans are spending far more on health care than ever before. In 1928–1929, total health care expenditures amounted to $3.6 billion, or less than 4 percent of the gross national product (GNP). By 1968–1969, they had risen to $60.3 billion, or nearly 7 percent of the GNP (12, p. 12). Public expenditures, greatly augmented after the adoption of the Medicare and Medicaid programs in 1965, were meeting 36 percent of the total in 1968–1969, while private insurance benefits, despite the fact that about four-fifths of the population had some insurance protection, were meeting only 22 percent (12, p. 12, and 13, p. 20).

What accounts for the sharp contrast between the high proportion of persons with some insurance coverage and the small proportion of total expenditures met by insurance benefits? The answer lies in the weaknesses of private health insurance protection: (1) provision for services in the hospital is much more common than for services in the physician's office or in the home; (2) there are limitations on reimbursable charges; (3) psychiatric care is covered only on a highly restricted basis; (4) dental care is barely beginning to be covered, although dental insurance protection is now spreading quite rapidly; (5) charges for health services are typically made on a fee-for-service basis, and increases in costs are passed on in the form of higher premiums; (6) hospital services are overutilized, except under prepaid comprehensive plans, partly because so many people have hospital insurance but no protection for care outside the hospital; and (7) despite much talk about the need for preventive care, insurance plans are poorly designed to encourage it.

THE PROBLEM OF RISING COSTS

Of the increase of nearly $50 billion in personal health care expenditures from 1928–29 to 1967–68, population growth accounted for 18 percent, increases in prices per unit of service for 38 percent, and all other factors, including an increase in the proportion of the

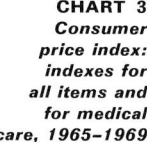

**CHART 3
Consumer
price index:
indexes for
all items and
for medical
care, 1965–1969**

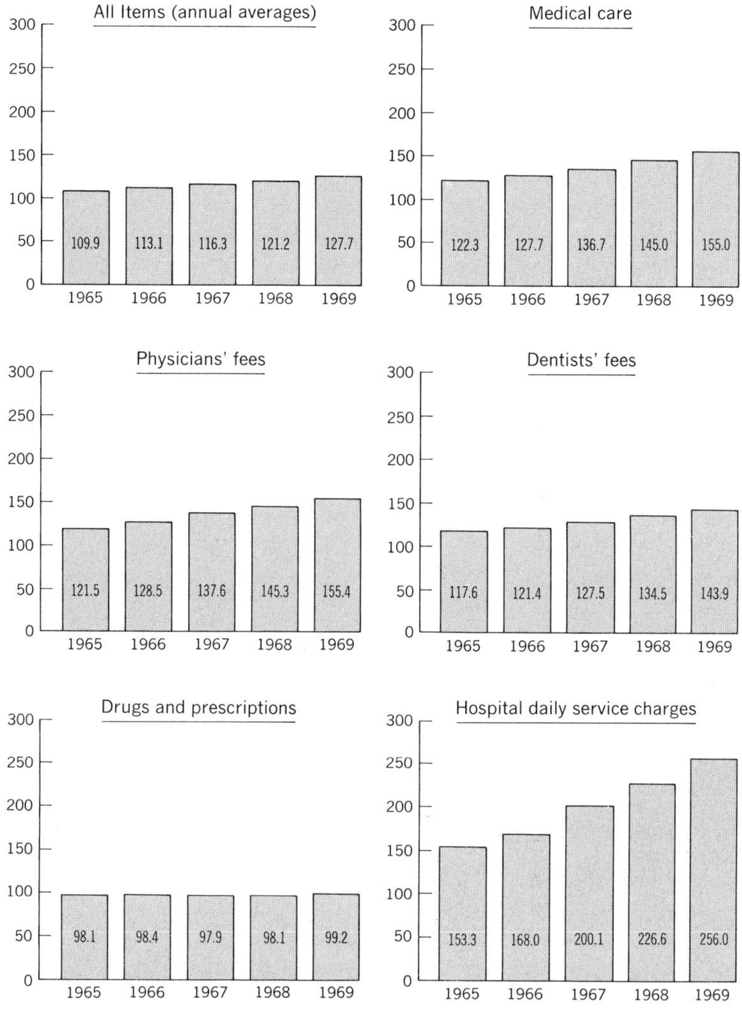

All Items (annual averages): 1965: 109.9; 1966: 113.1; 1967: 116.3; 1968: 121.2; 1969: 127.7

Medical care: 1965: 122.3; 1966: 127.7; 1967: 136.7; 1968: 145.0; 1969: 155.0

Physicians' fees: 1965: 121.5; 1966: 128.5; 1967: 137.6; 1968: 145.3; 1969: 155.4

Dentists' fees: 1965: 117.6; 1966: 121.4; 1967: 127.5; 1968: 134.5; 1969: 143.9

Drugs and prescriptions: 1965: 98.1; 1966: 98.4; 1967: 97.9; 1968: 98.1; 1969: 99.2

Hospital daily service charges: 1965: 153.3; 1966: 168.0; 1967: 200.1; 1968: 226.6; 1969: 256.0

SOURCE: U.S. Social Security Administration, *Medical Care Prices Fact Sheet, 1966–1969*, Research and Statistics note no. 2, February 23, 1970.

population receiving health care and the growing use of complex and expensive equipment, for 44 percent (14, p. 12). The rate of increase in the costs of health care rose sharply after Medicare and Medicaid came into effect (Chart 3). The effect of these measures was to expand the demand for health care by bringing it more readily within the reach of two needy and high-risk groups—the elderly and the poor, but the expansion occurred suddenly, in an industry in which the supply of both physicians and hospital capacity tends to be inelastic and to respond slowly to increases in demand. In addition, the expansion of demand encouraged long overdue increases in the compensation of nurses, other allied health workers, and hospital service personnel, who have traditionally been among the lowest-paid workers in the labor force.

The problem of inflation in the costs of medical care is going to be with us for a long time to come. Among the various ways of meeting the problem, overcoming shortages of health manpower and striving for greater efficiency in the delivery of health care are of paramount importance. They will receive major emphasis in this report.

SUMMARY   The crisis in the delivery of health care in the United States reflects the combined influences of five interrelated and overlapping factors: (1) unmet needs for health care, (2) rising expectations of the population for universal access to care, (3) critical shortages in, and inefficient utilization of, health manpower, (4) ineffective financing, and (5) rapidly rising costs.

3. The Scope of This Report

This report will be concerned primarily with the education of physicians and dentists and with the programs for training physician's and dentist's associates and assistants that are being developed in several university health science centers. The problems confronting medical and dental education are so broad in scope and so challenging that it would be impossible to deal with them adequately in this report if an attempt were also made to consider the education of all health personnel.

Shortages of nurses and allied health workers, as well as of physicians, are acute, and increased attention needs to be paid to the development of training programs for new types of health personnel. The Commission recognizes the importance of these problems, and in its report *Quality and Equality: Revised Recommendations, New Levels of Federal Responsibility for Higher Education*[1] it has recommended greatly expanded federal aid for higher education which will benefit students enrolled in nursing and allied health programs in all institutions of higher education, including comprehensive colleges and community colleges, which are playing increasingly important roles in the training of health personnel. In addition, our forthcoming report, *New Students and New Places,* will devote considerable attention to the changes that are occurring in the education of nurses and allied health workers.[2]

Throughout this report, a distinction is made between health care education and health care delivery. The Commission has not studied and is not competent to make recommendations about the

---

[1] This is a supplement to the Commission's first report, *Quality and Equality: New Levels of Federal Responsibility for Higher Education.*

[2] The forthcoming report of the National Commission for the Study of Nursing and Nursing Education (W. Allen Wallis, Chairman), summarized in reference 15, deals extensively with the problems of nursing education.

most suitable patterns of health care delivery. But it emphasizes that adequate health care education, while a prerequisite to adequate health care delivery, by no means guarantees it. No matter how many health professionals are trained, and no matter how adequately medical education facilities are distributed throughout the nation, Americans will not receive adequate health care unless a system is developed to deliver health care to those who need it, regardless of income, geographic location, age, or race. Unless health education efforts are coordinated with changes in the existing pattern of delivery of health care, the Commission's recommendations will not have maximum impact upon the actual health of Americans.

4. Medical Education Today

THE 60 YEARS SINCE FLEXNER

The famous Flexner report, issued in 1910, led to pronounced changes in medical education and in the quality of medical care in the United States. Briefly, it developed the themes that (a) medical care must be based on thorough knowledge of the biomedical sciences, (b) only high-quality medical schools should receive accreditation, (c) these schools should emphasize both laboratory work and extensive clinical experience, (d) the many inadequate proprietary medical schools which flourished in that period should be closed down, and (e) medical schools should be affiliated with universities (16).

The primary thrust of the post-Flexner development in medicine was the recognition of a scientific base in the natural sciences as a *sine qua non* for rational diagnosis and therapy. The reservoirs of scientific knowledge were in the universities, and, as a result, medical schools and teaching hospitals became more closely integrated with academic disciplines on the campus. This development was greatly encouraged following World War II by the expansion of federal expenditures for biomedical research from less than $50 million to about $1,200 million a year, with about $350 million of the latter amount going to medical schools. From the research-oriented university medical centers have come new knowledge and techniques which have revolutionized the control of disease within a single generation.

The university medical centers have become loci of sophisticated diagnosis and treatment. Their influence extends to the practitioners of the surrounding communities, resulting in a general increase in the quality of health care in the areas. But the centers' effect on the quality of care in their communities is far less significant than it could be if an effective health care delivery system became a primary element of medical center concern.

DOCTORS, DENTISTS, AND THEIR ASSISTANTS

One inescapable consequence of greatly increased medical knowledge and technology has been rapid specialization of health care personnel. Not only have professional health care workers become increasingly specialized, but they have steadily become a relatively more significant component of the labor force. In 1967, about 3,400,000 civilian workers were employed in health care (17, p. 8). Professionals constituted about 45 percent of the total, while nonprofessionals, including clerical workers and service workers in particular, were scattered through many other major occupation groups. Physicians (including osteopaths) constituted just about one-tenth of all health workers in 1967. A useful classification of health care jobs is presented in Table 2, but it excludes nearly 600,000 workers in health services who could not be identified in the 1960 Census occupational classification.

By 1969 women constituted about four-fifths of all persons employed in health services industries, largely reflecting their overwhelming predominance in nursing and some of the other allied health professions. But they were *not* well represented among physicians and dentists. Only about 6 percent of all physicians and surgeons and only about 8 percent of all medical students are women. This situation is in marked contrast to that in Western Europe, where in all countries women represent a considerably larger percentage of the medical profession than in the United States—for example, 30 percent in Germany and 20 percent in the Netherlands (18, p. 198). The representation of women in dentistry is even more limited—only 1 or 2 percent of American dentists are female (19, pp. 1–2).

Increasing the proportion of women in medical and dental schools, in the absence of other changes, would not increase the supply of physicians' and dentists' services, since many married women in these professions who have young children work only part-time or drop out of the labor force entirely.[1] But women are particularly well suited to serve as family physicians, pediatricians, psychiatrists, and in certain other specialties. The serious deficiency of child care centers in the United States is undoubtedly one of the factors that keeps women out of medical and dental schools, and out of professional practice later on.

Members of minority groups are also well represented only in the

---

[1] Among female medical school graduates active from 1931 to 1956, 45 percent were working full-time or part-time in 1964 (20, p. 491).

TABLE 2 Estimated employment in health care jobs, by level of job content and occupation, 1960

Health care job	Employment Number	Percent
High level		
Psychiatrists and neurologists	11,185	0.6
Physicians and surgeons (M.D. and D.O.)*	222,567	11.0
Dentists	86,887	4.3
Veterinarians	15,205	0.7
Life scientists—health	13,208	0.5
Podiatrists	7,600	0.4
Biophysicists	962	†
Biochemists	5,625	0.3
Administrators—hospital and other health institutions	12,000	0.6
Psychologists—clinical	5,888	0.3
Optometrists	16,205	0.6
Pharmacists	92,233	4.5
Health education specialists	1,000	0.8
Sanitary engineers	5,266	0.3
SUBTOTAL	495,791	24.4
Middle level		
Social workers, psychiatric	7,189	0.4
Social workers, medical	4,467	0.2
Chiropractors	13,853	0.7
Rehabilitation counselors	3,000	0.1
Speech and hearing therapists	6,200	0.3
Sanitarians	11,000	0.5
Industrial hygienists	1,300	0.1
Physical therapists	9,000	0.4
Occupational therapists	8,000	0.4
Other therapists	5,368	0.3
Medical laboratory technologists-technicians	53,720	2.6
Dietitians and nutritionists	26,470	1.3
Medical record librarians	8,000	0.4
Medical x-ray technicians	55,386	2.7
Dental laboratory technicians	19,711	1.0
Opticians, lens grinders, and polishers	20,406	1.0
Nurses, professional	581,289	28.6

TABLE 2
Estimated employment in health care jobs, by level of job content and occupation, 1960 continued

Health care job	Employment	
	Number	Percent
Dental hygienists	9,855	0.5
Midwives	896	†
SUBTOTAL	845,510	41.5
Low level		
Dental assistants, dental office	36,662	1.8
Medical office assistants	35,508	1.7
Medical record technicians	23,000	1.1
Practical nurses	207,966	10.2
Attendants, hospitals and other institutions	391,136	19.3
SUBTOTAL	694,272	34.1
TOTAL	2,035,573	100.0

*Excludes psychiatrists and neurologists.
† Less than 0.05.
SOURCE: J. H. Weiss, "A Job Classification for Health Manpower," *Health Services Research,* Spring 1968, pp. 48–64.

lower echelons of health manpower—chiefly in service occupations. Notable exceptions are Japanese-Americans and Chinese-Americans who have entered the higher ranks of the health professions to a significant extent. Although more than 11 percent of the nation's population is black, less than 2 percent of American physicians are black (21, pp. 1–2). In 1969, only 2.8 percent of all M.D. candidates were black (22, p. 1), and the majority of the black medical students were enrolled at Howard University and Meharry Medical College. Although 54 medical schools had special programs to recruit black students, the programs were held back by lack of adequate financial assistance for the students and by lack of funds for special efforts to overcome the academic deficiencies of some of these students (23, pp. 96–100). However, many of the leading medical schools are vigorously recruiting extremely able black students who are not in need of remedial academic programs.

The situation in dentistry is very similar. In 1965 less than 2 percent of all dentists were black, and in 1969 only 2 percent of all dental students were black. Only 21 of the 50 dental schools, other than Howard and Meharry, had any black students, and most of these had only one (24, p. 78).

The need to train more minority-group physicians and dentists is crucial. They can play a leadership role in stimulating more emphasis on adequate health care services and health education for minority groups, and they can undoubtedly relate to patients of their own races more effectively than white practitioners.

Medical education is very costly for students, regardless of race. They must meet tuition and subsistence expenses through, typically, four years of undergraduate premedical education and four years of M.D.-candidate education. Then, during the subsequent year of internship and three to five years of residency, their earnings are far less than these highly educated students would be capable of earning in regular jobs. Thus foregone earnings are high over a period of some 12 to 14 years. In view of this, it is not surprising to find that medical students are likely to come from families in the middle and upper-middle income brackets. In 1967, 63 percent of all medical students reported that they came from families with incomes of $10,000 or more. Only 48 percent of all families with heads aged 45 to 54—the age group in which medical students' parents are most likely to be found—reported that much income (25).

Dental education is about as costly as medical education but not nearly as prolonged. Thus total costs and total foregone earnings are considerably lower in the case of dental students.

[illegible]ements in adequate healthcare services and health education in minority groups, and they can undoubtedly [illegible] patterns of [illegible]

[illegible]

5. The Future of Health Care Delivery

Future changes in medical and dental education must be geared to impending changes in patterns of health care delivery. Although there is disagreement about the precise nature of the changes that are likely to occur, there is agreement that change is inevitable and imperative, and there is some consensus about its general outlines.

1. There will be a spread of prepaid group practice plans, such as Kaiser-Permanente plans, Detroit's Community Health Association, New York's Health Insurance Plan, the Group Health Cooperative of Puget Sound, and others. The Kaiser plans encourage preventive services by making a variety of them, including multiphasic screening and regular, periodic physical examinations, readily available. Members are either not charged for office visits or, at most, pay a nominal registration fee. There is a wide variety of specialists on the Kaiser staffs so that members are assured prompt attention by appropriate professionals. These physicians are all in group practice and are not compensated on a fee-for-service basis (26). Thus there are no incentives for excessive use of physician's or hospital services.

2. There will be much greater emphasis on achieving effective functioning of true health care teams in which the physician or dentist is at the center of the team and the work of allied health personnel is subject either to his direct or indirect supervision.

3. There will be a shift to greater emphasis on care outside the hospital in a wider variety of health care facilities than has been available. Neighborhood health clinics, facilities for ambulatory care of convalescing patients, and homemaker services to facilitate care in the home are all needed. There has been an encouraging beginning in the development of such facilities and services in the

1960s, but the movement is in its infancy and requires rapid expansion.

4 Gradually we are likely to shift toward a situation in which health care is a public utility. The government's role in protecting the health of the population will inevitably become broader in scope. In an era of increasing concern for the environment, greater attention will be paid to preventive epidemiology, population problems, control of water and air pollution, environmental sound levels, and related problems. As the trend toward a more comprehensive national health insurance system continues, the federal government will become increasingly concerned with adequacy and efficiency in the delivery of health care, with terms and methods of payment, and with the education and utilization of health manpower.

5 The rate of acquisition of new knowledge and technology in the biomedical sciences will continue to be impressive. Progress in diagnosis and therapy, involving increasingly complex facilities, as well as trained technicians and retrained physicians, will continue at a rapid rate. Perhaps the most important impact on the health care system will come from more extensive use of computers and automation techniques in institutional administration and patient care facilities.

Information networks will make possible the transmission of medical records for analysis and consultation without regard to geographic location. New therapeutic techniques will require new technologies, new kinds of trained personnel, and cooperation of many individuals as a closely integrated unit. Organ transplantation has been the subject of great public interest in the last few years, and intensive care units, hemodialysis, and high-intensity radiation therapy will become increasingly common.

As a result of the tremendous progress that has been made in overcoming and, in many cases, eliminating sources of acute illness, concern has shifted to the prevention of disease, diagnosis and treatment of degenerative diseases, and mental illness. Each of these will be affected by major developments in the next few decades.

The rate of advance of knowledge and technology is so rapid that physicians and other health professionals must remain students throughout their professional careers or face partial obsolescence in five to ten years. Expanded continuing education programs for physicians and other health workers, which are increasing in availability and quality, will be essential if optimum health care is to be provided.

6 The education, service, and research functions of medical and dental schools will become more effectively oriented to the shift from a *nonsystem* to a *system* of health care delivery.

The nation's goal should be adequate and effective health care for the entire population, regardless of income. Many of the recommendations that will be made in this report—for example, the provision of 9 new university health science centers, the development of about 126 area health education centers, and provision for a national health service corps—should help to overcome the present maldistribution of health manpower. Physicians, dentists, and allied health workers are likely to be attracted to areas where there are well-developed area health education centers. Our proposal, which calls for a broad geographic distribution of such facilities, should go far toward achieving more equitable geographic distribution of health manpower. Health personnel may be more willing to practice in remote, rural areas if there is a health education center within a reasonable distance. However, the full effect of such centers in attracting health manpower will doubtless not be experienced until a national health insurance system, perhaps with built-in features to provide special financial and nonfinancial incentives to health personnel for locating in remote areas, becomes a reality. A national health service corps could also play a key role in bringing health personnel to areas now poorly served.

6. The Future of Health Manpower Education

THE EVIDENCE OF A SHORTAGE OF PHYSICIANS AND DENTISTS

An extensive series of reports and special studies in recent years have projected shortages of health care personnel, especially of physicians (27, pp. 135–138; 11, vol. 2, p. 243; and 28, chap. 4). Some observers, however, dispute the existence of a current or impending shortage of physicians. They argue that the real problem is the maldistribution and inefficient use of physicians. They also argue that (1) the ratio of other health workers to doctors and dentists is increasing rapidly, (2) the work of the health care team will soon be far more effectively coordinated than at present, and (3) physician's associates and assistants with less prolonged training than the fully certified doctor now receives will increasingly take over some of the physician's duties so that his time will be released for the use of his highest skills.

The Commission has carefully considered these arguments. It agrees that these changes are occurring and will undoubtedly be accelerated during the 1970s, but we do not believe they will take place rapidly enough to rule out the probability of continuing shortages throughout this decade. We fully support the efforts to develop training programs for physician's associates and assistants, but these programs are just beginning and cannot possibly have much impact on the shortage of physicians before the end of the 1970s. In addition, it is altogether unrealistic to suppose that practicing physicians, especially those in the middle and older age brackets, are going to change their patterns of practice or their locale suddenly and drastically in order to overcome problems of inefficient utilization and geographic maldistribution of physicians. These problems will be overcome as more young doctors complete their medical education, as financing mechanisms are designed to overcome the shortages of health manpower in low-income areas, and as more vigorous efforts are made to achieve greater efficiency in the use of health manpower.

Whether or not one accepts as accurate the estimate of a current shortage of 50,000 physicians, cited by Dr. Egeberg, there is no question, in our judgment, that an *acute shortage exists*. One indication of it is the uneven geographic distribution of physicians discussed earlier. Another takes the form of long waiting lines for emergency services in hospital outpatient clinics. Another is the very long working week of the typical physician—for all reporting physicians, the median work week in 1968 was 60 hours (29, Table MD-9). In addition, the presence of large numbers of foreign medical graduates in the United States, especially among house officers (interns and residents), indicates that we are not training enough doctors.[1] In 1967 there were about 46,000 graduates of foreign medical schools in the United States, representing about 15 percent of all physicians. Approximately 19,000 of these worked in private practice, 14,000 as house officers, and nearly 9,000 as full-time medical staff of hospitals.[2] In recent years, many of these foreign graduates have come from relatively underdeveloped countries in which the quality of medical education is greatly inferior to the best medical training available in this country.

Although pressure to discourage the employment of foreign medical graduates from relatively underdeveloped countries may increase, it does not appear likely that such pressure will soon reverse the present trend toward increasing employment of physicians from abroad, at least as long as shortages of doctors in the United States continue. Yet it is widely regarded as an unsatisfactory solution of the United States physician shortage and is resented abroad as a "brain drain." Looking toward the future, the United States should become a net exporter of medical manpower, as part of the effort to raise the quality of medical education and medical care in underdeveloped countries. For similar reasons, more emphasis in American health science centers on research on diseases prevalent in underdeveloped countries is needed, and foreign students should be encouraged to enter United States medi-

---

[1] This is not to suggest that there is a clear-cut cause-and-effect relationship between the shortage of physicians in the United States and decisions of foreign medical graduates to come here. Many are attracted by the quality of our internship and residency programs.

[2] The remaining foreign medical graduates were chiefly medical school faculty members, administrators, or in research.

cal schools or to come here temporarily for training at the house officer stage, even if we eventually overcome the need to import them on a permanent basis.

The shortage of student places in United States medical schools, in relation to applicants, is such that the schools accepted only 52 percent of all applicants in 1967–68, and this ratio has not varied greatly for a number of years (29). As a result, many students go abroad for their medical education. About 11 percent of all American M.D. candidates attend foreign medical schools and, on their return, are among the foreign medical graduates appointed as interns and residents (although those who attend Canadian schools are not classified as foreign medical graduates). Until the number of entrant places in United States medical schools has expanded sufficiently to permit acceptance of a considerably larger proportion of applicants, medical students will continue to seek admission to foreign medical schools.

For all these reasons, the Commission believes that strong support must be given to expansion of the number of student places for M.D. candidates in medical schools as well as to the newly developing and innovative programs for the training of physician's associates and assistants. The great majority of experts on medical education who have been consulted in the preparation of this report agree.

On the whole, there is less evidence of a shortage of dentists than of physicians, *in relation to current demand.* However, dentists are unevenly distributed geographically (Chart 2), and unmet need is particularly acute in low-income areas. But dentists' hours of work tend to be much shorter than physicians' hours, averaging 43.2 hours a week in 1964 (30, p. 8). Moreover, very few foreign dental school graduates are employed in United States dentistry.

As in the case of physicians, it is very difficult to estimate the ratio of dentists to population that might be "adequate" in 1975 or 1980. Dentists' productivity has been rising steadily and, in the absence of an accelerated increase in the per capita demand for services, one would expect the ratio to decline. But the per capita demand for services may increase, not only because of the spread of privately financed dental care plans, but also because of such possibilities as a federal program to ensure dental services for children or eventual inclusion of dental care in a national health insurance system.

Existing projections of the demand for dentists are based on maintaining the existing ratio of dentists to population and take no account of either an accelerated increase in demand, on the one hand, or a change in the rate of increase of productivity on the other (31). There has been an accelerated increase in dental school places in recent years, and estimates provided by the Council on Dental Education of the American Dental Association project an increase from 4,430 dental school entrants in 1970–71 to 5,400 in 1980–81. These projections have been used in estimating the cost of the federal aid to dental students and their institutions recommended in this report. The Commission believes that at least the expansion of dental school places indicated by these projections is needed.

Dental education is considerably less prolonged than medical education. Most dental schools require only two or three years of college education as a prerequisite for entry, although the proportion of entrants who have received a bachelor's degree has been growing and amounted to 59 percent of the total in 1968 (32, p. 16). As compared with M.D.'s, relatively few dental students go on beyond the four-year D.D.S.-candidate program to undertake advanced education in dentistry, but the proportion is increasing, and in 1968–69 about 10 percent of all dental school students were enrolled in advanced education courses (32, pp. 12 and 25).[3]

Despite the current progress in dental productivity, even more rapid progress could be achieved through more extensive use of dentist's assistants and dental hygienists and through greater emphasis on preventive programs. The view has been expressed that "dentistry has an excellent chance of being the first health profession to become truly preventive" (33, p. 9). Several other countries, notably New Zealand, have achieved impressive results through programs designed to ensure that all children receive dental care (34).

THE EXPANSION OF HEALTH MANPOWER EDUCATION

The Commission believes that vigorous efforts should be made in the 1970s to induce expansion of student places for M.D. and D.D.S. candidates in university health science centers and that these centers should also develop and expand programs for the training of physician's and dentist's associates and assistants.

The armed services have effectively used practically trained physician's assistants—the medical corpsmen, and there is growing interest in the development of programs for the education of phy-

[3] The data do not include students in dental hygienist, dental assistant, and continuing education courses.

sician's associates and assistants in civilian life. A program for the training of physician's assistants at Duke University Medical Center has been underway for five years. Its students are recruited from those with previous health care experience, either as medical corpsmen or in civilian life as practical nurses. The course is two years in length and leads to a certificate (35, p. 151). For the last several years the University of Colorado School of Medicine has had a pediatric nurse practitioner education program and is now training at the bachelor's and master's level a new kind of pediatrics associate (36). Pediatrics lends itself particularly well to the use of associates, since so much of pediatric practice consists of routine checkups and treatment of minor illnesses.

Also of great interest is the Medex program at the University of Washington School of Medicine—a program specifically designed to take advantage of the training and experience of ex-military corpsmen, who are given three months of training at the medical school, followed by a year of preceptorship (a kind of apprenticeship) as assistant to a physician. The program is funded on a research and demonstration basis by the National Center for Health Services Research and Development (NCHSRD), and several replications at other institutions are now being supported. However, the Center cannot provide training funds as such because funds available for health manpower training are limited to specified occupational categories. The NCHSRD regards the Medex program as a promising model for the training of physician's assistants and estimates that, from about 30,000 corpsmen discharged each year, of whom about 10 percent are qualified at the independent-duty level of responsibility, and also from previously discharged corpsmen, approximately 3,000 independent-duty ex-corpsmen a year could be recruited for Medex programs (37 and 38).

There are now more than 40 programs for the training of physician's assistants and similar types of auxiliary personnel, while 66 programs for the training of pediatric nurse practitioners are in operation or in some stage of development. The majority of these programs are of very recent origin and are in comprehensive colleges or community colleges, but, according to the head of the health services manpower section of NCHSRD (38):

Because of the especially close and personal relationship of this mid-level worker to the physician, we are loath to see the rapid proliferation of this type of training outside of substantial medical centers, with the exception of the preceptorship training which we believe can best be given by the physician who will ultimately employ him.

Programs such as these are clearly in an experimental stage, as NCHSRD recognizes, but their graduates are in great demand, and they offer promise as a way of augmenting the supply of medical personnel, especially in small towns and rural areas, where the supply of general practitioners has been declining sharply as older men die and young doctors do not appear to take their places.

In 1968-69, 259 dental assistants were being trained in dental schools (32, p. 12). D.D.S. candidates are trained to work with them in dental school, with the result that when dentists enter practice they have experience in the most effective ways of using assistants. This type of experience should also be part of the M.D.'s education.

There is also considerable interest among medical educators in greater emphasis on the training of primary or family physicians, but many educators believe that the predominant trend will continue to be toward the provision of primary physician care by internists, pediatricians, and obstetricians. In line with this development, there should be increased emphasis, eventually encompassing all medical schools, on training associates and assistants for these three groups of specialists. But we also recognize that other types of allied health personnel not now envisioned may be developed and that the shape of medical health teams in the 1980s and the 1990s cannot be reliably predicted today. Meanwhile, as the Thirty-seventh American Assembly pointed out, there is an urgent need for modifications of licensing and legal liability provisions to permit effective utilization of physician's associates and assistants "while assuring quality of services" (39, p. 6).

There is also a need for more dental schools to experiment with and develop programs for the education of dentist's associates and to expand their existing programs for dental assistants. As we move toward provision of dental care on an insured basis, dentists will be hard pressed to meet the increased demand, and many more dentists are likely to seek the services of dentist's assistants and dental hygienists. Although many dentists use such assistants, the overall ratio of assistants to dentists in dental offices was only 1.35 per dentist in 1965 (30).

The Office of Health Planning of the University of California has prepared for the Carnegie Commission a number of alternative projections of the increase in the number of physicians per 100,000 population to the year 2002, based on differing assumptions with respect to the annual increase in the number of entrants to United

States medical schools. Three of these projections are included in Table 3.[4]

In view of the comparative stability of the physician-population ratio prior to the 1960s, the rapid increase in this ratio indicated by all these projections may seem surprising. There are two main reasons for it: (1) as the number of medical school graduates increases to a level well beyond that prevailing in the recent past, the number of graduates will exceed by large margins the number of physicians dying or retiring, and (2) the population is not expected to increase as rapidly in the next three decades as in the 20 years or so following World War II.

The Commission believes that projection C is based on an attainable and desirable estimate of the annual increase in the number of medical school places to about 1978. In fact, progress has been so rapid in the last few years that the number of entrants in the fall of 1970 is likely to exceed the 10,800 indicated by projection C.

Whether the number of medical school entrants should be expanded after 1978 is a question that cannot be answered at the present time, since it is impossible to predict the number of M.D.'s per 100,000 population that will be "adequate" in relation to the very different supply and demand situation which may prevail in the 1980s. On the one hand, we expect the increase in demand to rise sharply, particularly if a national health insurance system becomes effective. On the other hand, physician productivity may rise at an accelerated rate in the 1970s as increasing use is made of various substitutes for physicians. The net effect of these opposing trends in the next decade cannot be reliably predicted. Toward the end of the 1970s, the question of any additional increases in medical school entering places should be reappraised.

It is sometimes noted that the ratio of physicians to population in the United States is higher than in many other countries, including some that have a superior ranking in terms of life expectancy or infant mortality, and that the ratios indicated by the projections in Table 2 for 1977 or 1982 might well prove to be excessive. However, it must be kept in mind that the proportion of physicians en-

[4] A monograph providing a detailed explanation of the methodology of these projections, prepared under the direction of Dr. Mark S. Blumberg, formerly Director of Health Planning, University of California, will be issued by the Carnegie Commission. It should be noted that the definition of physicians used in preparing the projections differs from the definition (all nonfederal physicians) in Chart 2.

TABLE 3 Projections of number of physicians per 100,000 population, based on three alternative projections of number of medical school entrants, United States, 1967–2002

Year	Medical school entrants*			Active physicians (M.D. and D.O.) per 100,000 population†		
	A	B	C	A	B	C
1967	9,479	9,479	9,479	146.8	146.8	146.8
1968	9,863	9,863	9,863			
1969	10,200	10,200	10,200			
1970	10,800	10,800	10,800			
1971	11,400	11,400	11,400			
1972	12,000	12,000	12,000	153.9	153.9	153.9
1973	12,500	12,500	12,900			
1974	13,000	13,000	13,800			
1975	13,500	13,500	14,700			
1976	14,000	14,000	15,300			
1977	14,500	14,500	15,900	161.4	161.4	161.4
1978	15,000	15,000	16,400			
1979	15,000	15,500	16,800			
1980	15,000	16,000	17,100			
1982	15,000	16,000	17,700	168.8	168.9	171.3
1987	15,000	16,000	19,200	175.3	177.0	182.1
1992	15,000	16,000	20,400	180.7	184.3	194.2
1997	15,000	16,000	21,400	183.4	188.5	205.0
2002	15,000	16,000	21,600	185.8	192.4	216.4

*Excludes entrants to osteopathic medical schools.
† Assumes 13,000 foreign medical school graduates will permanently enter the United States between 1968 and 1977, but none will enter permanently thereafter. Excluded from the data are 10,500 foreign medical graduates in the United States in 1967 who were judged to be here temporarily. However, some temporary foreign medical school graduates are assumed to be in the United States in all subsequent years, although they are not included in the ratios above.
SOURCE: Office of Health Planning, University of California.

gaged part-time or full-time in research and the proportion in military service outside national boundaries are undoubtedly higher for the United States than for most other countries.[5]

It is extremely difficult to predict the rate of increase of physician's and dentist's associates and assistants likely to be trained in university health science centers. For purposes of estimating the

[5] Recent comparative data indicate that eight countries—Australia, Austria, Czechoslovakia, Denmark, West Germany, Hungary, Israel, and the U.S.S.R.— had higher ratios of physicians to population than the United States (2, pp. 857–858).

cost of federal aid which we recommend for such programs, we project a gradual rise from about 500 students in 1970–71 to 3,500 in 1979–80. This projection could turn out to be excessively optimistic or seriously deficient, depending on the speed with which university health science centers develop such programs and the extent of aid available from federal and other sources. Despite the previously mentioned NCHSRD estimate that 3,000 independent-duty ex-corpsmen a year could be recruited for Medex programs, we do not believe it is realistic to predict that university health science centers will develop and expand programs rapidly enough to absorb such large numbers of ex-corpsmen for some time to come.

The acceleration in the increase of entrant places in both medical and dental schools in recent years has clearly been stimulated in large part by increased federal aid, especially in the form of construction grants. Similarly, much of the projected expansion for the 1970s is dependent on federal construction funds and will not be forthcoming in the absence of adequate appropriations. Recently, the appropriations have fallen considerably below amounts authorized by Congress.

The Commission believes that the number of medical school entrants or their equivalent should be increased from the 10,800 estimated for 1970–71 to about 15,300 by 1976 and to about 16,400 by 1978. The desired increase of 5,600 new places—52 percent—for medical school entrants by 1978 can be achieved in three ways:

1   If all existing medical schools shifted from four- to three-year programs between the B.A. and M.D. degrees by 1973–74, as suggested subsequently in this report, the estimated number of places for new students could be increased, without incurring construction costs, by about 4,500 more entrants by 1976–77—31 percent more than estimated for the latter year.

2   Existing schools can also add new places by physical expansion. The smaller and developing schools in particular may be expected to increase their average class size to at least 100 and, in some cases, to 200 or more. With physical expansion of present schools, places for new entrants could easily be increased by at least 8 to 13 percent, and potentially by much more.

3   Establishment of nine recommended new schools will provide perhaps 900 to 1,350 new places for entrants, an additional increase of 8 to 13 percent.

Thus acceleration of instruction and physical expansion of existing and developing schools can increase new places by 39 to 43 percent, and new schools can provide the balance in realizing a 52 percent increase in new places for medical school entrants. Some experts argue that expansion should be confined to existing medical schools—on the ground that expanding existing institutions is less costly than building new ones. However, the statistical evidence does not altogether support this view, since expansion of existing schools has frequently required the replacement of old, outmoded buildings at high cost. Moreover, the Commission believes that new university health science centers are needed to achieve adequate geographic distribution of such facilities. The case for broad geographic distribution rests primarily on the role we envisage for university health science centers in improving the quality of health care in the areas in which they are located. They will play an important role in augmenting the supply of health manpower in their areas, in part through their power to attract house officers (interns and residents) who are likely to practice there later, and in part through the role we believe they should play in stimulating and guiding the training of allied health personnel in nearby comprehensive colleges, community colleges, and high schools. However, in view of the interstate mobility of medical school graduates, broad geographic distribution of M.D.-candidate education may not in itself lead to a more even geographic distribution of physicians per capita. Financial and nonfinancial incentives to encourage physicians to practice in deficit areas are also likely to be needed.

The American Medical Association and the Association of American Medical Colleges have also called for rapid expansion of medical school entrant places and have been helpful in providing the Carnegie Commission with recent unpublished data on medical school expansion. The joint AMA-AAMC statements on health manpower of March 5, 1968, and April 16, 1968, are included in Appendix A.

The Commission recommends that the number of medical school entrants should be increased to 15,300 by 1976 and to 16,400 by 1978. Toward the end of the 1970s, the question of whether the number of entrant places should continue to be increased will need to be reappraised. The expansion in the number of medical school entrants should be accomplished through an average expansion of about 39 to 44 percent in existing and developing schools by 1978, with nine new schools accounting for about 900 to 1,350 entrant places, adding another 8 to 13 percent. The number of dental school entrants should be increased at least to 5,000 by 1976 and to 5,400 by 1980.

We also recommend that all university health science centers consider the development of programs for the training of physician's and dentist's associates and assistants, where they do not exist, and that, wherever feasible, such programs be initiated forthwith. The Commission recommends, also, that in developing their plans for expansion, university health science centers should adopt programs designed to recruit more women and members of minority groups as medical and dental students.

In addition, the Commission recommends the conversion of schools of osteopathy to schools of medicine, wherever feasible.

THE ROLE OF UNIVERSITY HEALTH SCIENCE CENTERS

The Commission believes that university health science centers should be responsible for the education of health care personnel and for cooperation with other community agencies in improving the organization of health care delivery. These centers should cooperate with comprehensive colleges, community colleges, and high schools in planning and evaluating training programs for allied health workers who will be educated in these institutions. An important function of the university health science centers, in cooperation with professional associations in their areas, should be continuing education for all health manpower occupations.

All university health science centers need not conform to a single model. Some will continue to be leading centers for biomedical research, but even though every center needs a research program to fulfill its educational function, not all of them should seek to develop extensive research programs. Medical and dental students do need to understand research procedures and methods, however, so that they will be prepared as practitioners to interpret reports on new research and so that they will have a thorough understanding of the contributions of research (as well as an understanding of its limitations) to improved practice.

Some university health science centers, like Case Western Reserve, will be leaders in curriculum reform and innovation (40). Others, like Harvard and Johns Hopkins (which are also leaders in research), will develop community experiments in health care delivery and financing systems. But all will need to broaden their faculties to include social scientists who have the training to analyze the social and economic aspects of medical and dental care.

Both the education and research programs of medical and dental schools need to be broadened to include concern with needed improvements in health care delivery and with changes occurring in patterns of health care—such as group practice and prepaid health plans. This will require closer relationships between the health science centers and social science departments on main university campuses as well as with organizations and individuals in local communities.

Many of the most important innovations in the delivery of health care have been developed outside the universities by such agencies as the Kaiser Foundation on the West Coast, the Health Insurance Plan of Greater New York, and similar organizations. Closer relationships between university health science centers and these organizations would be highly desirable. Indeed, it is highly important that a genuine two-way relationship develop between university science centers and the communities adjacent to them. The health science centers can be a significant influence for improving the quality of health care and health manpower education in an area but should also be *responsive* to ideas and suggestions developed by community groups.

In the past, university health science centers and their parent universities have not considered improvement of the quality of health care in their areas as *primary goals*. We are pleased to note that several medical schools have recently taken important steps in this direction. America's land-grant institutions have been responsible for remarkable advances in agriculture and the quality of rural life. Although they now tend to be philosophically remote from such a concept, university health science centers could well play a similar role in urban life. Social concern, especially among students, favors this attitude, so the time may be right for university health science centers to meet the challenges of helping communities develop model health care systems throughout the nation.

Every health science center should encompass university activities related to the education of physicians, dentists, and other health professions. It should be capable of handling the most complex and sophisticated medical problems. It should serve as the coordinating hub and reservoir of expertise for a system of institutions that may include area health centers, neighborhood health centers, rural clinics, hospitals, group practice organizations, and medical societies.

Although teaching hospitals affiliated with university health science centers will perform important activities of the centers, there is no need for a teaching hospital to be owned by a health science center. In fact, a center that is not involved in the complex problems of owning a teaching hospital will have advantages over those that do.

<u>The Commission recommends that university health science centers should be responsible, in their respective geographic areas, for coordinating the education of health care personnel and for cooperation with other community agencies in improving the organization of health care delivery. Their educational and research programs should become more concerned with problems of health care delivery and the social and economic environment of health care. All new medical and dental schools should be parts of university health science centers, and, wherever feasible, existing separate medical and dental schools should likewise become parts of university health science centers.</u>

ACCELERATION OF MEDICAL AND DENTAL EDUCATION

Many experts on medical and dental education believe that the entire period of education, especially for the medical students, is much too long. It is costly for the students, costly for the schools, and costly for agencies that provide student support.

The Commission believes that acceleration efforts are essential and structures its recommendations for federal aid in this report to stimulate it in medical and dental education. At the same time, we believe that a broad liberal arts education is essential for professionals in the health field and do not favor acceleration at the *expense* of an adequate liberal arts background. Consideration should be given, however, to the fact that students typically enter college today with more high school preparation in the humanities and the social sciences than was true several decades ago. They are also exposed to television and other communications media from an early age and tend to be far more aware of social, political, and economic problems than was formerly the case.

There are a number of ways in which the length of medical education could be reduced. These include: (1) straightforward revision of the curriculum for M.D. and D.D.S. candidates so that the required courses could be completed in a three-year period; (2) provisions for advanced standing for students entering with extensive premedical or predental preparation; (3) providing instruction for M.D. and D.D.S. candidates during all or part of the summer; (4) reducing the total number of years required for premedical and medical education combined or for predental and dental education combined; and (5) eliminating the internship year, which is now indistinguishable from a residency year, since it also involves specialization. The American Medical Association approved elimination of the internship in June, 1970. Effective July 1, 1975, no internship will be approved unless it is integrated with a residency.

If all medical schools were to move from a four-year to a three-year program between the baccalaureate and M.D. degrees, the size of each class could be increased by nearly one-third without increasing the total number of students enrolled at any one moment of time and without requiring additional physical facilities. Since the training would be more intensive, additional faculty members would still be required, but substantial savings would nevertheless be possible. Nearly two-thirds of the construction costs needed to achieve a 52 percent increase in new student places if the four-year programs were continued would be saved by program acceleration. There might also be savings of up to one-third in operating expenses. Institutional cost per students would decrease by about one-third, and a similar reduction in the total amount needed for student assistance would be possible. Clearly, also, the students' loss of foregone earnings would be reduced, and the supply of physicians and dentists could be increased more rapidly if the total duration of the students' education could be reduced.

Savings may also be realized by accelerating programs during the residency period, but they will not be as dramatic as those effected in the years between the B.A. and M.D. and D.D.S. degrees.

Accelerated programs of medical education are in effect at Case Western Reserve, the University of Minnesota, the University of Nebraska, the Medical College of Ohio (Toledo), Ohio State, Temple, the University of Texas (Galveston), and the University of Washington. Dartmouth and Michigan State are shifting from a two-year program, after which a student has been obliged to transfer to a four-year medical school, to a program in which an M.D. can be obtained in three years. At Stanford, where the curriculum is individualized and highly flexible, it is possible for a student to graduate in considerably less time than the conventional four years. Yale also has an individualized and flexible curriculum. The California College of Medicine at the University of California, Irvine, is one of three medical schools now beginning freshmen classes in July, rather than September, in order to accelerate the medical training program. Other acceleration programs are under consideration.

A proposal for pronounced acceleration has been developed at the University of Michigan but not as yet adopted. Premedical and medical education would be treated as an integrated unit, with a substantial reduction in the number of years required to obtain both the baccalaureate and M.D. degrees. Students completing the first few years of the program would have the option of shifting to one of a number of biological fields rather than going on to the clinical portion of the program (41).

<u>The Commission recommends that all universities with health science centers develop plans for accelerating premedical and medical education. The Commission also recommends that plans be developed for shortening the total duration of predental and dental education where it is unnecessarily prolonged. We particularly favor a program calling for three years (instead of four) after the B.A. to obtain the M.D. or D.D.S. and a three-year residency (instead of the typical four years of internship and residency).</u>

INTEGRATION OF THE CURRICULUM

A number of universities have adopted or are developing plans for restructuring preprofessional and professional education in the health sciences. The plans differ somewhat in their objectives, but several of them would result in acceleration of premedical and medical education as well as in consolidation of all instruction in the basic sciences on main university campuses.

The Michigan proposal, discussed above, emphasizes integration of the premedical and medical curricula along with a sharp reduction in the total duration of premedical and medical education.

Harvard and the Massachusetts Institute of Technology are considering a proposal for a joint Harvard–M.I.T. School of Health Sciences and Technology, offering a program emphasizing courses in human biology and leading to a master's degree. Graduates would be qualified to enter medical school or to go on for a Ph.D. in the biological sciences, in the natural sciences, or in engineering as these subjects relate to biology, or in the social sciences as they relate to health, and to enter appropriate levels of teaching (42).

The Illinois Board of Higher Education recently approved a plan for reorganization of the College of Medicine at the University of Illinois, which, among other changes, would establish two types of schools: (1) schools of basic medical sciences at the Medical Center campus in Chicago and at the university's Urbana-Champaign campus and (2) schools of clinical medicine. The schools of basic medical sciences will promote basic knowledge and understanding of sciences relevant to preparation for careers in dentistry, medicine, nursing, pharmacy, and associated medical fields. It is anticipated that the typical basic science curriculum for medical students will be one year in duration.

The schools of clinical medicine would offer students transferring from the basic science schools a three-year curriculum to complete the work for the M.D. degree (43). One of the clinical schools would include the regular faculty and clinical departments of the present College of Medicine based at the University of Illinois hospital in Chicago. Thus the structure of medical education would resemble that in Britain, where instruction in the basic sciences is given at Oxford, Cambridge, and other universities, followed by clinical instruction in hospitals in London and elsewhere. Plans are being developed for the establishment of a second school of clinical medicine in the Chicago area. Additional clinical schools in Peoria and Rockford are now in the development stage (Appendix B, Table 1).

A somewhat similar plan has been in effect at Indiana University for some time.

These plans, in differing ways, involve integration of instruction in the basic sciences in a program which could lead to entry into medical school for clinical instruction in what has conventionally been the second or third year of the M.D. candidate's education or could lead to work for the Ph.D. in biological or other sciences related to health. The Michigan proposal would treat premedical and medical education as an integrated curriculum.

At the University of California School of Medicine, San Diego, the academic master plan allocates some medical school faculty positions to other campus departments for individuals whose scientific interests are related to medicine and human biology. These departments occupy space in the School of Medicine and in return accept teaching responsibilities within the medical curriculum. The curriculum is divided roughly into the first, or basic sciences, year; the second, or medical sciences, year; the third, or clinical sciences, year; and a fourth year of electives. But integration of instruction in the basic and clinical sciences is sought by including clinical correlatives in the first two years and basic science correlatives in the last two years (44, p. 64).

An obvious advantage of shifting instruction in the basic sciences out of the medical schools and on to main university campuses is the probable increase in overall student-faculty ratios in premedical and medical education in the basic sciences that would result. Medical schools tend to have very low student-faculty ratios, averaging 3.9 students per full-time faculty member in 1968, if all M.D. candidates and postgraduate medical students are included, and 1.6 students per full-time faculty member if only M.D. candidates are included (45, pp. 1558 and 1561). These ratios may be compared with an overall ratio for higher education of about 13 full-time-equivalent students per full-time-equivalent faculty member, but it must be kept in mind that the overall ratio includes community colleges, where faculty members are not engaged in research. In universities, and especially in medical schools, many faculty members spend a good deal of time on research. The ratio of graduate students to faculty in universities generally would be more nearly 6 or 8 to 1.

Objections have been raised to some of these proposals on the ground that they would conflict with a trend toward integration of instruction in the basic and clinical sciences and would not meet the strong desire of many medical and dental students for contact with patients early in their medical or dental education. However, if the plan involves integration of preprofessional and professional education, with an appreciable shortening of the period preceding clinical instruction, this objection is less valid. It would also appear to be less valid if the basic sciences program involves emphasis on human biology, as in the Harvard–M.I.T. proposal. In addition, opportunities can be created for early clinical experience through part-time or summer jobs for medical and premedical students in university health science centers and area health education centers.

However, in view of the various conflicting considerations, some universities are considering experimenting with variations of this type of change. The Johns Hopkins School of Medicine, for example, is giving consideration to transferring some, but not all, of the training in the basic sciences to the main university campus.

Also under consideration at Hopkins is the "possibility of creating a College of Medical Sciences that would take in at an earlier age all those interested in the health sciences. A broadly oriented core base of varying complexity and subsequent multiple-track options would allow final differentiation of nurses, radiobiologists, research scientists, and physicians" (46, pp. 32–33). This general concept is receiving increasing attention and needs more emphasis in the health manpower curricula of comprehensive colleges and community colleges as well as in universities. Among other things, it might help to reverse the current trend toward proliferation of professional health workers' associations defined, like the traditional craft unions, on a narrow specialty basis.

The Commission believes, also, that as medical and dental curricula are reformed and accelerated, there is a strong case for awarding a master's degree at an appropriate stage, probably following completion of the basic science curriculum, as proposed for Harvard and MIT.

However, the student who receives a master's degree or completes the program at an existing two-year medical school, such as the schools at Brown University and the University of Hawaii, sometimes has difficulty in being admitted to another medical school to complete his M.D.-candidate program. The Commission believes that such two-year schools should be converted to provide full M.D.-candidate education as soon as possible and that no new two-year medical schools should be established unless they lead on to M.D.-candidate education within the same university system.

In connection with the integration of university curricula in the health sciences, the Commission also believes that new schools of public health should be parts of university health science centers and that existing schools of public health should become parts of health science centers wherever feasible. With their emphasis on the prevention of disease, public health programs would contribute to greater emphasis on prevention within the health science centers.

The Commission recommends that all universities with health science centers, and especially those developing new centers, consider plans for (1) greater integration of preprofessional and professional curricula, (2) increasing the student's options so that basic training in health-related sciences can lead on to training for a variety of health-related professions as well as medicine and dentistry, (3) awarding a master's degree at the end of this basic training period, and (4) integrating instruction in the basic sciences on main university campuses if this can be accomplished without major costs associated with the shift, without interfering with integration of basic science and clinical science instruction, and without delaying the opportunities for students to have early contact with patients.

In addition, the Commission recommends that existing two-year medical schools that do not lead on to M.D.-candidate education within the same university system be converted to provide full M.D.-candidate education as soon as possible and that no new two-year schools of this type be established.

The Commission also recommends that new public health schools be made parts of university health science centers and that existing public health schools become parts of such centers as soon as possible.

The Commission recommends that new university health science centers consider providing clinical instruction in selected hospitals on the British model.

OTHER CURRICULUM REFORMS

The Commission believes that many of the reforms in medical and dental education increasingly being sought by students deserve serious consideration. Students are calling for more flexible admission standards to bring in applicants with varied educational and cultural backgrounds. They want students to be represented on admissions committees and to be given more opportunities than they now have to influence the curriculum. They believe that a larger proportion of the curriculum should be elective and that there should be more chance for independent study activities and individualized instruction. And, as previously mentioned, they are calling for early contact with patients and for more carefully integrated relationships between basic science and clinical instruction so that abstract parts of the curriculum become more meaningful in relation to the treatment of individual patients. They seek less compartmentalized instruction and more emphasis on comprehensive medicine, with the patient viewed as an individual in a family and in an environmental situation that may have an important bearing on his condition.

In addition, the Commission believes that medical students should be given more training than they now receive in the problem of alcoholism and in the growing problem of drug addiction.

The Commission also believes that, along with abolition of the internship, as already suggested, many changes are needed in graduate medical education. The deficiencies in residency training were clearly identified in the report of the Citizens Commission on Graduate Medical Education, which stressed among other things the need for (1) a more carefully integrated program for the resident, (2) responsibility of the entire faculty, rather than of individual departments, for continuous planning and evaluation of residency programs, and (3) the establishment of a permanent commission on graduate medical education for the purpose of planning, coordinating, and periodically reviewing standards for graduate medical education (47). There is also a need for providing a broader educational experience for the resident. In the teaching hospital, he tends to see acutely ill individuals, frequently with unusual conditions. He also needs experience that would come from periods spent in community hospitals, neighborhood clinics, convalescent facilities, and, where feasible, in doctors' offices.

<u>The Commission recommends that all university health science centers give serious consideration to curriculum reforms. Their admission policies should be made more flexible and their programs more responsive to the expressed needs of students. Greater emphasis should be placed on comprehensive medicine in both the M.D.-candidate program and in graduate medical education. In all phases of medical and dental education, including residency programs, there should be more careful integration of abstract theory and clinical experience. Residency programs should be planned and reviewed by the entire faculty, and residency training should include experience in community hospitals, neighborhood clinics, and other facilities, as well as in teaching hospitals.</u>

THE LOCATION OF NEW UNIVERSITY HEALTH SCIENCE CENTERS

The Commission believes that there should be a university health science center in every metropolitan area with a population of 350,000 or more, except for those areas which can benefit from the impact of centers that already exist in other geographically convenient communities. The Commission has identified eight metropolitan areas of at least this size and an additional metropolitan area, Duluth-Superior, with a population falling somewhat below 350,000, in which we believe university health science centers should be established (Table 4). Duluth-Superior is located so far away from the nearest medical school (in Minneapolis-St. Paul) that its needs cannot be adequately served without a university health science center of its own. Moreover, a university health science center in the Duluth-Superior area would serve large parts of northern Minnesota, Wisconsin, and Michigan.

Not included in Table 4 are 27 communities, many of them with a population of 350,000 or more, that have medical schools in the development stage. These developing schools are included, along

TABLE 4
Carnegie Commission goals for new university health science centers by 1980 (not including medical schools in development in 1970)

Standard metropolitan area	Estimated population, July 1, 1967 (in thousands)	Percentage increase in population, 1960–1967
Phoenix, Arizona	859	29.5
Norfolk-Portsmouth, Virginia	646	11.7
Springfield-Chicopee-Holyoke, Mass.*	557	4.6
Jacksonville, Florida	505	10.8
Wilmington, Del.-N.J.-Md.	481	16.0
Tulsa, Oklahoma	451	7.8
Fresno, California	416	13.6
Wichita, Kansas	396	3.7
Duluth-Superior, Minn.-Wis.	273	—1.4

*Metropolitan state economic area.
SOURCE: U.S. Bureau of the Census, *Current Population Survey: Population Estimates*, ser. P-25, no. 411, Washington, D.C., 1968; and American Medical Association, *Medical Education in the United States, 1968–1969*, Chicago, 1969. Information on medical schools that have begun development since publication of the latter volume has been supplied by the Council on Medical Education of the AMA.

with existing university health science centers and recommended new health science centers, on Map 1 and in Appendix B, Table 1.

The Commission recognizes that plans are being formulated for new medical schools in some of the communities in Table 4 as well as in other communities not included. However, we believe that, for communities with populations below 350,000, the area health education centers suggested in the following section would be a more appropriate solution.

The Commission also recognizes that local initiative is desirable, and usually essential, in planning for a new university health science center. In the absence of local initiative, it may be difficult to develop centers in the nine communities we have identified.

The Commission recommends the development of nine new university health science centers.

THE ROLE OF AREA HEALTH EDUCATION CENTERS

In some parts of the country the distances between university health science centers are likely to be very great, as in the sparsely populated mountain states. Elsewhere, concentration of people in congested urban areas would overwhelm the facilities of even the largest health science center. In both types of areas there should be "area health education centers," which would provide facilities for patient care, often on a referral basis from surrounding areas; educational programs for house officers and, to some extent, for M.D. candidates who could rotate through an area health education center from a university health science center; clinical experience for allied health students; and continuing education programs for health manpower.

These area health education centers, in essence, would be satellites of the university health science centers and would be visited on a regular basis by the faculty of the health science centers with which they were affiliated. Their educational programs would be developed and supervised by the health science faculty, and their patient care functions would rely on the expertise of the health science center personnel. The area centers in turn would provide assistance and counsel to the community and neighborhood health care facilities, including the private practitioner.

There are examples of existing institutions, including the Mary I. Bassett Hospital in Cooperstown, New York, which are serving such functions in their areas. In a somewhat different category is the Mayo Clinic in Rochester, Minnesota, if only because its reputation is such as to draw referral patients from all over the country. It trains about 700 residents in every specialty, is affiliated with the University of Minnesota Medical Center, and is developing plans for an M.D.-candidate program.

There are other examples of cooperative efforts to raise the quality of care in areas remote from university health science centers. These include Bingham Associates, centered in Boston, but carrying out field work throughout Maine; the Duke Foundation, which has funded a program to improve the quality of care in rural hospitals in North Carolina and South Carolina for 35 to 40 years; and a system of cooperative hospitals in the state of Wisconsin.

The nucleus of an area health education center would be a hospital, usually a community hospital, but perhaps in some cases a Veterans' Administration hospital. The house officers at the hospital would receive instruction from the faculty of the medical school with which the center was affiliated, in most cases on a visiting basis, but there would be a need for a small group of faculty members permanently located in the center to plan and administer both the educational programs for the house officers and continuing education programs for physicians and other health workers in the surrounding area. M.D. and D.D.S. candidates would receive part of their clinical instruction in such centers on a rotating basis. Within the hospital, or adjacent to it, there would have to be office space for faculty members and other administrators of the educational programs as well as classrooms. Like the university health science centers, the area centers should cooperate with comprehensive colleges and community colleges in the area in planning curricula for allied health workers.

The functions of area health education centers would be as follows:

1 To maintain a community hospital of outstanding quality, many of whose patients would be admitted on a referral basis from smaller communities in the surrounding area

2 To conduct educational programs under the supervision of the faculty of the university health science center with which the area center is affiliated

3 To have these educational programs include

   a Residency programs

   b Clinical instruction for M.D. candidates and D.D.S. candidates who would come there from the university health science center on a rotating basis

   c Clinical experience for students in allied health programs

   d Continuing education programs for health manpower in the area, conducted in cooperation with local professional associations

4 To provide guidance to comprehensive colleges and community colleges in the area in the development of training programs for allied health professions

5 To cooperate with hospitals and community agencies in the planning and development of more effective health care delivery systems

6 To conduct limited research programs concerned primarily with the evaluation of health care delivery systems

In some of the sparsely settled states, area health education centers would have to be affiliated with university health science centers in neighboring states with larger populations. These arrangements should be worked out on a regional basis, as suggested below in the section on regional planning.

The Commission recommends the development of area health education centers in areas at some distance from university health science centers which do not have sufficiently large populations to support university health science centers of their own, and in a few metropolitan areas needing additional training facilities but not full health science centers. These area centers would be affiliated with the nearest appropriate university health science center and would perform somewhat the same functions recommended for university health science centers, except that the education of M.D. and D.D.S. candidates would be restricted to a limited amount of clinical education on a rotational basis, and research programs would be largely restricted to the evaluation of local experiments in health care delivery systems.

THE LOCATION OF AREA HEALTH EDUCATION CENTERS

In developing its suggestions for the location of area health education centers, the Commission has carefully considered the following criteria: (1) distance from an existing university health science center, a developing center, or a recommended new health science center; (2) the population of the community and its surrounding area; and (3) the objective of providing for enough area centers so that no portion of a state or region would be remote from such a center. Nevertheless, in sparsely populated states the centers would inevitably have to be farther apart than in more thickly populated states.

The Commission believes that the final selection of locations for area health education centers should be based on careful regional planning. We are therefore *suggesting* the locations indicated by our analysis but are not firmly *recommending* them. However, we believe that the number of centers indicated by our analysis is probably quite close to the number that would be needed to provide adequate geographic distribution of such centers.

In addition to the criterion of geographic distribution, we have also applied a criterion of at least one university health science center or area health education center for every 1,500,000 persons in the larger metropolitan areas. On this basis, we are recommending the development of five area health education centers in the Los Angeles metropolitan area, one in the San Francisco–Oakland metropolitan area (in the East Bay), two in Detroit, one in Pittsburgh, and one in the New York metropolitan area.

The Commission is suggesting, in all, 126 locations for new area health education centers, indicated on Map 2 and listed in Appendix B, Table 1. The appendix table indicates where there is a Veterans' Administration (V.A.) hospital that is not affiliated with a medical school in a community for which an area health education center is suggested. However, the Commission does not believe V.A. hospitals would be appropriate as nuclei for area health education centers unless their policies were changed to permit the admission of patients of all types instead of veterans only. Under present policies, their patients are almost exclusively male and tend to be older persons suffering from long-term disabilities.

As the population grows and the centers develop, there may well be a case for converting some of these proposed area health education centers into university health science centers in the future.

We estimate that, if our recommendations for new university health science centers and suggestions for area health education centers are carried out, by 1980 about 95 percent of the population will be within no more than an hour's traveling time from a university health science center or an area health education center.

The Commission recommends the development of 126 new area health education centers, to be located on the basis of careful regional planning.

7. Financial Support and the Federal Government

The Carnegie Commission believes that medical and dental education are critically underfunded and that greatly increased financial support is required to bring about (1) the development of a sufficient and effective supply of physicians and dentists and their associates and assistants, (2) equality of opportunity to enter these health professions, (3) effective use of educational resources, (4) regional dispersion of health manpower educational institutions, (5) equitable distribution of the cost burden, and (6) adaptation of health manpower education to changing patterns of health care delivery.

To achieve these objectives will require that the federal government play a major role in the financing of health manpower education. The federal government collects about two-thirds of all tax revenues and is in a position to rely much more heavily on the personal and corporate income taxes than is feasible for state and local governments. Its tax structure is more equitable and more income-elastic, yielding revenues that rise relatively more rapidly than the GNP, whereas the sources of revenue generally available to state and local governments are less equitable and less income-elastic. Thus, as the economy expands, the federal government is in a much better position to increase its expenditures on public services.

Furthermore, as a result of the adoption of the Medicare and Medicaid programs, the federal government is now far more heavily involved in the financing of health care than ever before. Yet these programs are placing a major strain on the nation's inadequate supply of health manpower and health care facilities. There is the additional consideration that states with low per capita incomes encounter serious difficulty in providing the substantial funds needed for expansion of health manpower education, although, with their limited capacity to attract M.D.'s educated elsewhere, many of these states have developed more medical student places relative to their needs than some of the states with high per capita income.

The case for major federal financing is particularly strong in relation to M.D. candidates. Less than half of the graduates of United States medical schools are practicing in the state in which they received the M.D. degree, whereas well over half of those receiving residency training tend to practice in the state where they received that training (25). In other words, there is no very direct relationship between a state's investment in the education of M.D. candidates and the social return to the state. In view of this, there is considerable reluctance on the part of state governments to expand investment in the education of M.D. candidates. At the house officer level, the social return to the state can be more clearly demonstrated. This is also true of the education of allied health personnel, who are likely to be employed in the state in which they received their training.

Experimental programs for the training of physician's associates and assistants, though of much shorter duration, cost as much per student per year as the education of M.D. candidates, particularly in the early stages when classes are very small (35 and 38). Programs for dental assistants are also costly, partly because of the expensive equipment that must be used. Thus, if we are to expand the number of physician's and dentist's associates and assistants rapidly enough to have an appreciable impact on the productivity of physicians and dentists, a substantial federal contribution toward the cost of these programs is required. The federal aid for such programs and their students recommended in this report is confined to university health science centers or separate medical and dental schools. Programs for the training of physician's and dentist's assistants in comprehensive colleges and community colleges would be assisted by the federal aids to higher education recommended in the Commission's report *Quality and Equality: Revised Recommendations, New Levels of Federal Responsibility for Higher Education.*

In the years since World War II, the federal government has assumed major responsibility for providing funds for biomedical research. The Commission believes that this support should continue, but that the time has now come for an equally vigorous effort to expand the education of health manpower and to stimulate major changes designed to relate the future education of health manpower to probable changes in the delivery of health care.

Recently an HEW task force has called for direct federal aid to medical education and for the shifting of the responsibility for health manpower within the federal structure. On federal aid to medical education, the report said (48, p. 1):

> Because of a traditional reluctance to directly involve the federal government in the financing of medical school education, desperately needed financial support has been funneled through research grants to medical schools. While biomedical and clinical research conducted by the medical schools has been of great value and is an important element in attracting outstanding scholars and researchers, it is frequently a counter-productive incentive to improving the efficiency and teaching aspects of medical education. Therefore, support of the educational function should be separate and distinct from support of the research function. A more direct approach, depending on stipends to both the student and the medical school, would help reduce the financial burden of medical education for the student and provide the medical schools with positive financial incentives to increase their productivity.

A particularly urgent problem is the plight of medical schools, chiefly private institutions, which are in grave financial difficulties. A total of 61 medical schools have been awarded Special Projects Grants by the federal government on the basis of some condition of financial distress (49, p. 2), and in July, 1970, a bill authorizing $100 million in emergency aid to medical and dental schools "in financial distress" was passed by the Senate and sent to the House (50, p. 9).

The types of federal financial support recommended by the Commission include (1) student grants and loans, (2) institutional grants for educational expenses, (3) grants to university health science centers and university-affiliated area health centers for the advanced education of house officers, (4) grants and loans for construction, (5) start-up grants, (6) research grants, and (7) funds for manpower research and regional planning. The recommendations for grants to institutions are carefully designed to stimulate not only expansion of but also needed changes in health science education.

STUDENT GRANTS

In view of the high cost of medical and dental education, there is a particularly critical need for grants for students from low-income families who wish to undertake such education. The case for providing medical and dental education grants to students from low-income families also rests on the need to provide equal opportunity to students who are members of minority groups, since there are indications that reluctance to incur indebtedness for the financing of education may be particularly prevalent among such groups.

In the light of the substantial financial return to the individual who invests in medical or dental education, it is sometimes argued that assistance to the medical or dental student should take the form exclusively of loans. The Commission does not fully support this position, in view of the psychological barriers to incurring indebtedness on the part of students from low-income families, an attitude that is undoubtedly explained in part by the tendency for low-income families to experience income instability.

In view of the high cost of medical and dental education, the Commission recommends a maximum grant of $4,000 per year for medical and dental students, a larger amount than we have recommended for graduate students in higher education generally, partly because medical and dental students have less opportunity to work as teaching or research assistants. We do not agree with those who favor a maximum grant which would cover tuition at the individual's chosen school plus a subsistence allowance, on the ground that such a policy would encourage institutions to increase their tuition charges. As indicated below, the Commission believes that, in order to prevent an inflationary trend in tuition charges, university health science centers should be induced to adopt uniform tuition fees as a condition for the provision of federal cost-of-education supplements.

In determining the student's need, it will be necessary to derive a formula based on such factors as total family income over the past several years, total family assets, and the number and ages of children in the family. The income distribution of families with heads aged 45 to 54 is a more appropriate criterion for determination of the number of students potentially eligible for a grant than the income distribution of all families, since parents of medical and dental students are likely to be in that age group, and incomes of these families tend to be higher than those of families with younger or older heads. Median income for families with male heads aged 45 to 54 amounted to $10,940 in 1968. The median incomes for the first and third quartiles were $7,690 and $12,240, respectively. The Commission assumes that a maximum grant would often be necessary for students from families with incomes falling within the lowest fourth of this income distribution and that partial grants would be available for those in the next fourth, with more lenient criteria for students from large families.

The Commission recommends a federal program of grants in amounts up to $4,000 a year for medical and dental students from low-income families and for students from low-income families enrolled in associate and assistant programs in medical and dental schools.

STUDENT LOANS

Because medical education and dental education are expensive, and because medical education is exceptionally prolonged, only students from upper-income families are likely to be in a position to meet all the expenses of medical or dental education without the assistance of either grants or loans, and many students who are eligible for grants will also need to borrow funds. Indeed, a substantial percentage of all medical students now receive both grants and loans (25).

The Commission believes that the proposal for an Educational Opportunity Bank (EOB), as proposed by the report of the Panel on Educational Innovation to the U.S. Commissioner on Education and other federal officials (51) and by several independent economists, is particularly well suited to the financing of costs of medical and dental students. The returns to investment in education, especially for medical students, are high so that loan repayment obligations typically would not be burdensome. Under EOB proposals, a borrower would pledge a given percentage of his annual gross income for a fixed period of years after graduation. Thus, the amount repaid in dollars would vary directly with income. The plan would therefore involve an element of income redistribution and would provide a modest financial incentive for physicians and dentists to practice in areas where they could expect incomes below the average for their professions, since repayment obligations would likewise be lower.

The EOB would be a nonprofit agency established under the auspices of the federal government, with its capital made available by the United States Treasury through the sale of government bonds. The program would be administered through the institutions of higher education. There would be no income or means test as a condition of eligibility. Students could borrow a maximum amount equal to tuition plus a subsistence allowance (including dependents' allowances) plus necessary travel expenses for out-of-state students, *minus* any grant or fellowship stipends available to the student from any public or private source.

A medical student should be able to borrow funds for the full cost of his medical education in return for a pledge to pay 3 percent of his medical earnings in each of his first 20 years of professional practice (52). The Commission suggests a 30-year repayment period, which would require a lower percentage of earnings.

Married women with children of preschool age would be excused from repayment obligations during this period if they worked half-time, as an incentive to encourage their participation in the labor force.

> The Commission recommends an Educational Opportunity Bank for medical and dental students, including house officers, with repayment excused during periods of house officer training and during two years of military service.

A NATIONAL HEALTH SERVICE CORPS

The Commission believes that a national health service corps should be developed to bring improved health care service to low-income and rural areas of the nation. The time is right for such a development. Medical students and other students in the health professions are increasingly interested in problems of delivery of health care to the poor, and many are motivated to participate in neighborhood clinics or other facilities in low-income areas. Furthermore, the Administration's policy of withdrawing troops from Vietnam should result in a decreased level of military need for physicians. The normal period of service in the corps would be two years.

As a financial incentive for service in the corps, in addition to modest compensation, the Commission believes that loan repayments should be excused during periods of service and that, in addition, 25 percent of the maximum indebtedness that a student is eligible to incur would be forgiven. This would mean that, for M.D.'s with only small amounts of indebtedness, the entire debt would be canceled.

> The Commission recommends the development of a voluntary national health service corps. As an incentive for participation in the corps, an M.D. or D.D.S. would be excused from loan repayments during periods of service, and 25 percent of the maximum indebtedness he is eligible to incur would be forgiven.

TUITION POLICY

One of the arguments against an EOB program is that institutions would be encouraged to raise their tuition charges, once a student could be certain of borrowing the full amount of his tuition. The Commission believes that, as a logical corollary to assumption of major financial responsibility for the financing of medical and dental education by the federal government, a uniform tuition charge should be established for medical and dental education.[1] The charge would be adjusted from time to time to reflect changes in costs of education per student.

At present there are wide variations in tuition charges from institution to institution, but tuition charges tend to be quite high, particularly at private medical and dental schools. During the period 1957-58 to 1967-68, median tuition in public medical schools rose from $500 to $750, while median tuition in private medical schools rose from $1,005 to $1,920 (25). The federal aids proposed in this report would have the effect of making such wide variations unnecessary. Moreover, differentiation between residents and nonresidents of a given state would be inconsistent with the principle of major federal financing responsibility and with the goal of nationwide recruitment of students by the institutions and nationwide choice of institutions by the students.

In the absence of expanded federal aid, including the cost-of-instruction supplements recommended in this report, the trend toward higher tuition charges is certain to continue, especially in the private institutions. Somewhat ironically, also, the increases may have to be particularly large in the institutions that are in financial difficulties, since they tend to be especially dependent on tuition as a source of income.

If the student is required to pay high tuition over a prolonged period of M.D.- or D.D.S.-candidate education, it is readily apparent that the total cost is likely to be so high that many students will be faced with the unfortunate choice of abandoning medical or dental education or going very heavily into debt.[2] Yet for the institutions, the cost of both medical and dental instruction is very high. It is extremely difficult, however, to determine precise costs because the educational process is encompassed in a complex aggregate of teaching, research, and patient care functions. Yet the extent to which costs of research and patient care associated with the educational process are included in accounting of instructional costs

---

[1] The case for a uniform tuition charge is not as strong in other higher education programs, with the possible exception of education of Ph.D.'s, since the role of state governments in financing higher education is expected to be relatively greater than in the education of physicians, dentists, and Ph.D.'s, and states can be expected to vary greatly in their relative contributions to the cost of education for many years to come.

[2] Foregone earnings are also very high for medical and dental students, amounting to an estimated $8,750 a year (54).

varies greatly among institutions. There is a need for more careful studies of these elements of costs for accurate determination of educational cost per student.

Not only are costs of instruction in medical and dental schools high, but they vary widely among schools. On the basis of data from a number of studies, they may amount to at least $6,000 in a number of schools and exceed this amount in many, running as high as $15,000 or $16,000 in some of the leading medical schools. The Commission believes that tuition should represent only a relatively small proportion of this instructional cost and that the remainder should be met through federal support, state government support, and private endowment funds. The Commission is convinced that low tuition is likely to be more evenhanded in its impact than high tuition accompanied by a very complex package of grants and loans. Even if tuition is held to low levels, many students will have to meet the tuition charge through student aid and loans. All things considered, we suggest a uniform tuition charge of approximately $1,000 a year.

It should be emphasized that the cost-of-education supplements recommended below far exceed any loss in tuition which university health science centers would experience as a result of this policy.

The shift to such a uniform tuition policy would have to take place gradually. An abrupt shift would disrupt existing relationships among institutions in their capacity to attract students. Moreover, provisions of state law and, in some cases, of state constitutions would have to be changed to permit uniform tuition fees for nonresidents and residents of a state. Thus the Commission believes that provisions of federal legislation directed toward requirement of a uniform tuition fee should not become effective until four years after the effective date of the legislation and that, in the interim, institutions should shift toward such a policy as rapidly as circumstances permit.

The Commission recommends a relatively low uniform national tuition policy for institutions providing medical and dental education.

COST-OF-INSTRUCTION SUPPLEMENTS TO INSTITUTIONS

To ensure not only maintenance of current effort but also expansion and change in health science education, the Commission believes that a substantial program of cost-of-instruction supplements per student should be undertaken by the federal government. This approach to financial assistance to institutions to aid in meeting instructional costs is dependent upon the concept that *separate* national funding will continue to be provided for the research programs of these institutions and that patient care costs will be met, to a greater extent than at present in many teaching hospitals, by insurance or by such programs as Medicare and Medicaid.

Institutions would not, however, receive these instructional supplements automatically. The federal agency charged with the responsibility of administering the grants should negotiate with each institution to make certain that it is developing plans not only for the expansion of medical and dental education but also for their greater effectiveness and efficiency. In addition, the institution should be required to:

1 Use the funds for instructional costs and not for other purposes
2 Initiate the steps necessary for a gradual shift to the uniform tuition policy recommended above and for the elimination of admission requirements favoring residents of the state
3 Refrain from discrimination on the basis of race, creed, or sex and also pursue positive policies to encourage the admission of members of minority groups

In addition, the federal government should take into account whether each state is meeting its share of the costs in comparison with other states (Table 5, section 8).

Federal payments to institutions would be available in the following amounts:

1 An amount equal to the institutions' enrollment of students working toward the M.D. or D.D.S. or enrolled in a physician's associate or assistant program, multiplied by $4,000. This amount is not by any means intended to cover the full instructional costs per student. As suggested above, these costs vary from an estimated $6,000 to $15,000 or $16,000. The Commission believes, however, that the institutions should continue to receive part of their support for instructional costs from other public (state) or private sources.
2 In addition, an amount equal to that portion of the enrollment of students in the above programs in excess of enrollment in the fall of 1970, multiplied by $4,000. These bonuses would be available for a total period of eight years following initiation of a substantial program of expansion by an institution, designed to achieve an increase of at least 20 percent in first-year student places within a

period of four years. Moreover, every institution should be expected to increase its average class size to at least 100.

Payment of the supplements would not begin until actual entry of additional students and would be based on the number of such entrants enrolled in a given year. If a university health science center had initiated a significant expansion plan for added student places at any time from 1967 through 1970, the bonuses would be available for the added students for the remainder of the eight-year period. The Commission believes that even though the expansion should be accomplished within a four-year period, higher costs would be incurred for as long as eight years—hence the stipulation that the bonuses should be available for eight years.

<u>The amounts in 1 and 2 above should be adjusted for medical and dental schools with three-year programs to enable those schools to receive the same amount of institutional aid as they would if they were four-year schools. This adjustment should be made until about 1980 but then should be reviewed.</u>

3 An amount equal to the total number of house officers in university health science centers and in university-affiliated hospitals or area health education centers, multiplied by $2,250, provided that no individual house officer shall be counted for more than three years, and provided that a policy is in effect to encourage specialization in fields in which a shortage exists and discourage it in fields in which there is a surplus, such as surgery. These supplements should also be paid under the condition that the institution make an effort to reduce the duration of house officer education and make it more effective. As indicated above, the internship year is being eliminated in medical education, and the Commission believes that it should not be replaced by an *additional* year of residency.

4 As an incentive for *major* curriculum reform, additional cost-of-instruction supplements of $2,000 a year per student enrolled in M.D.- or D.D.S.-candidate programs, in physician's or dentist's associate or assistant programs, and, under specified conditions, in the last year of premedical or predental programs, for up to three years. These bonuses would be available for the following types of changes:

   a Introducing physician's or dentist's associate or assistant programs, with the bonuses to be available for such programs for a period of three years even if they had been initiated before the effective date of the legislation, but only for the number of students enrolled in these programs

b   A program for major curriculum reform designed to provide greater efficiency, effectiveness, and flexibility in premedical and medical education or in predental and dental education, along the lines of proposals and plans discussed in the section on "integration of the curriculum" in this report

If the program is designed to achieve a reduction in the total duration of preprofessional and professional education, the number of bonuses would be based on the total number of students enrolled in M.D.- or D.D.S.-candidate programs and in the last year of preprofessional education. These bonuses would also be available for the number of postbaccalaureate students enrolled in integrated basic science programs designed to prepare a student to enter what is now the third year of a medical or dental school, as in the University of Illinois schools of basic sciences. The bonuses would not be provided for a program to reduce the length of M.D.- or D.D.S.-candidate education from four to three years without any other major change, since schools with three-year programs would be entitled to receive the same amounts under paragraphs 1 and 2 above as if they had four-year programs.

All the cost-of-instruction supplements recommended above would be based on the number of full-time-equivalent students rather than on the number of full-time students, as under the Health Manpower Act of 1968. This change would be designed to encourage schools to permit students to enroll on a part-time basis—a policy which might make it possible for some married women with young children to enter or complete their medical or dental education.

The Commission recommends (1) cost-of-instruction supplements to university health science centers for each medical and dental student enrolled; (2) bonuses for expansion of enrollment; (3) cost-of-instruction supplements to university health science centers and their affiliated hospitals for each house officer; and (4) bonuses for curriculum reform. The supplements and bonuses would also be available for each student enrolled in physician's and dentist's associate and assistant programs as well as for students in the last year of premedical or predental education if curriculum reform is designed to achieve a reduction in the total duration of preprofessional and professional education.

CONSTRUCTION GRANTS AND LOANS

Construction funds should be allocated for new and expanding university health science and area health education centers and for renovation and replacement of existing buildings, with the federal government providing up to 75 percent of the total cost of construction in the form of grants and making available 25 percent in the form of loans, if the institution chooses to apply for a loan. These funds would also be available for separate medical or dental schools.[3] The Commission believes that the present maximum federal contribution of 50 percent of construction costs is inadequate since institutions experience serious difficulty in obtaining the other 50 percent from public or private sources.

Since federal construction funds will inevitably be limited in relation to total sums involved in all applications, the allocations process should consider steps being taken by the institution to undertake curriculum reform, to implement the other policies recommended in this report, and to achieve maximum effectiveness and efficiency. Preference should be given to institutions that, among other things, plan new facilities involving innovations effecting lower building costs and more flexible interiors. In other words, the allocation process should encourage competition among institutions in meeting these objectives.

START-UP GRANTS

In view of the high costs associated with the developmental stage of a new university health science center and with the acquisition of land, especially in central city areas, the Commission believes that start-up grants should be made available for nonconstruction costs of new university health science centers. These funds should be provided for centers in the development stage by 1970 as well as for the nine new centers recommended for development during the 1970s. Funds would be made available from the time of issuance of a "certificate of reasonable assurance." As in the case of construction grants and loans, the start-up grants should be allocated on a competitive basis to ensure maximum effectiveness

---

[3] The construction grants and loans would be available for facilities which are primarily for teaching purposes but which might also be used for research purposes or for medical or dental library purposes, as provided by the Health Manpower Act of 1968.

and efficiency in the curriculum. The grants should not exceed $10 million per center.

The Commission recommends (1) construction grants for university health science centers and area health education centers in amounts up to 75 percent of total construction costs, with the remaining 25 percent available in the form of loans; and (2) start-up grants for new university health science centers in amounts not exceeding $10 million per center.

SUPPORT OF RESEARCH

The Commission believes that a vigorous biomedical research program is essential for continued progress in combating disease and that it is an integral component of the process of medical and dental education. Our recommendations above for cost-of-instruction supplements to support this educational process are predicated on the continuation of federal support for biomedical research and for studies of the needed changes in health manpower education and in the delivery of health care.

It is the view of the Commission that the total amount provided to university health science centers for research by the federal government should be maintained at its current percentage of the GNP (0.042 percent). Changes in appropriations to reflect changes in the GNP should be made on the basis of a moving average of the total GNP in order to avoid abrupt or irregular shifts in amounts. Federal allocations for research should cover the full costs of research projects, since present requirements for institutional contributions frequently result in a diversion of funds from instructional and other expenses. The Commission recommends that not less than 10 percent and not more than 25 percent of the research grants to any university health science center take the form of institutional grants rather than grants for specific research projects.

The Commission recommends that federal financial support of research in university health science centers be maintained at its present percentage of the GNP; that funds should be made available to support research on methods of achieving greater efficiency in health manpower education and in the delivery of health care as well as for biomedical research; that federal allocations should cover the total cost of research projects, and that not less than

10 percent and not more than 25 percent of the research grants to any university health science center should take the form of institutional grants rather than grants for specific research projects.

NATIONAL AND REGIONAL PLANNING

The Commission believes that existing federal legislation providing for regional, state, and local planning of health services should be strengthened and expanded. The legislation providing for Regional Medical Programs (Public Law 89-239 of 1965) was designed to ensure that the results of research relating to cancer, heart disease, strokes, and related diseases were made available in the treatment of the victims of these diseases. It provides funds for planning the expansion and improvement of appropriate treatment centers in existing hospitals and other health care facilities and for continuing education of physicians. The results have been encouraging in some parts of the country, although there is evidence that more progress has been made in relatively small communities and rural areas than in urban areas, especially in the ghetto areas of large cities (53). The legislation requires the representation of medical schools on regional advisory committees, and in a number of cases university medical centers have fiscal responsibility for the programs.

Also operating through state and local agencies is the Comprehensive Health Planning program authorized through Public Law 89-749 of 1966. The CHP agencies bring together at the state and local levels representatives of providers of medical care and of consumers to develop plans for filling gaps in available services and eliminating duplication and overlapping of services.

The Commission believes that existing legislation should be strengthened and expanded to provide for regional planning relating to (1) the location of health manpower educational institutions and (2) the expansion of and improvement in the delivery of all types of health care, including preventive care. One of the purposes of the strengthened legislation would be more adequate regional planning of appropriate locations for neighborhood health centers.

One of the most difficult concepts to comprehend is what constitutes a "region." . . . It is unfortunate that "geography" or boundaries should have played so dominant a role in the early discussions of what constitutes a region. Experience will indicate that a region can best be defined by reviewing the functional relationships that exist within any given area (55, p. 14).

The Commission believes that revised federal legislation should provide for studies designed to develop more appropriate identification of regions suitable for health planning. In sparsely populated areas of the country, a region might include several states. For example, under the auspices of the Western Interstate Commission on Higher Education, which includes all the Western states, a plan has been developed to design and implement a cooperative program to improve health care through medical education in the states of Idaho, Montana, Nevada, and Wyoming. Where such regional planning bodies in higher education already exist, they might well be incorporated in a federally supported regional health planning program, but other groups of sparsely settled states which have no such mechanism at present should be identified.

The strengthened regional planning legislation should also provide funds for broad programs of continuing education of physicians and other health personnel rather than the current limited programs for heart, cancer, and strokes. In fact, some of the regional planning bodies have developed programs that cover medical care more broadly. The Commission believes, also, that the present planning structure, comprising Regional Medical Programs, Comprehensive Health Planning agencies in the states, and separate provisions for the allocation of funds for hospital construction under the Hill-Burton Act is unduly complex. There should be a single group of regional planning agencies, which would develop plans in cooperation with state and local governments, university health science centers, area health education centers, and professional associations. Federal funds should be allocated to these regional planning bodies to cover 50 percent of the costs of continuing education programs, with the remainder to be met from other public and private sources, including professional associations. To the extent that costs are covered by fees paid by physicians and other health manpower personnel, they should be deductible from federal and state income taxes.

In connection with these regional planning activities, the university health science centers should have central responsibility for planning and coordinating all regional educational programs for health manpower, in cooperation with all the other agencies and institutions concerned, including professional associations. The central responsibility for planning changes in the delivery of health *care,* however, should be in the hands of regional agencies, in cooperation with state and local agencies, and with private institutions, including group health plans. But there should be very close relationships between the university health science centers and the agencies responsible for problems of health care delivery. The goal should be adequate and effective delivery of health care in all parts of the nation as well as broad geographic distribution of health manpower educational institutions.

The Commission recommends the strengthening of existing federal legislation for regional, state, and local health planning to encompass regional planning of all health manpower education and health care facilities. The university health science centers, along with their affiliated area health education centers, should have central responsibility for the planning of health manpower education, while the central responsibility for planning changes in the delivery of health care should be in the hands of regional agencies, in cooperation with state and local agencies, as well as appropriate private institutions. Continuing education of health manpower should be a major concern of the university health science centers and area health education centers with federal funds providing 50 percent of the financial support of such programs.

RECERTIFI-CATION In view of the rapid rate of progress of medical and dental knowledge and the associated problem of educational obsolescence of practicing physicians and dentists, the Commission recommends the development of national requirements for periodic reexamination and recertification of physicians and dentists. These functions should be carried out by specialty boards and other appropriate bodies, such as the Board of Family Physicians, which has adopted requirements for periodic reexamination and recertification. Among other advantages, such requirements would provide a powerful stimulus to participation in continuing education programs and to the expansion of existing efforts of professional associations to encourage continuing education.

The Commission recommends national requirements for periodic reexamination and recertification of all physicians and dentists by specialty boards and other appropriate bodies.

STUDIES OF HEALTH MANPOWER The Commission believes that there is a critical need for continuous studies of growth and change in health manpower, analyses of future supply and demand and of the productivity of health manpower, and research on the development of new allied health specialties. Present federal programs relating to health manpower research are seriously inadequate. Augmented funds should be provided for more comprehensive studies of health manpower, both within the federal government and through research grants to university health science centers and appropriate university research institutes. The program should be centered in the Department of Health, Education, and Welfare but should be conducted in close cooperation with the broader manpower studies of the Department of Labor.

<u>The Commission recommends expansion and strengthening of the health manpower research programs in the Department of Health, Education, and Welfare, in cooperation with the Department of Labor, to encompass broad continuous studies of health manpower supply and demand. Research funds should be made available for specialized studies of these problems in university health science centers and appropriate university research institutes.</u>

A NATIONAL HEALTH MANPOWER COMMISSION

The Commission believes that the time has come for appointment of a National Health Manpower Commission to make a thorough study of changing patterns of utilization of health manpower, with particular reference to the development of new types of allied health personnel, including physician's and dentist's associates and assistants. The National Advisory Commission on Health Manpower submitted an extensive and authoritative report in 1967 (11), but its estimates of future supply and demand were limited to physicians, dentists, and nurses and were concerned only with the period to 1975. In view of the rapid development of training programs for various types of physician's assistants just in the last few years, an extensive and authoritative study of these programs and their future potential is needed, along with studies of the training and use of other novel types of allied health personnel.

The work of the proposed commission should include careful analysis of changing patterns of health care delivery, including the growth of prepaid health plans and group practice, and of the probable impact of various proposals for national health insurance on health care delivery. It should also encompass changes occurring in institutional arrangements for the education of health manpower, including the shift in the training of nurses and other allied health workers from hospitals to comprehensive colleges and community colleges.

The Commission also believes that the proposed commission should make a thorough study of existing problems in the licensing of health manpower personnel and should investigate the feasibility of a national licensing system. Such a national system might be developed under the leadership of the federal government but with the active participation of the American Medical Association, the Association of American Medical Colleges, the American Association of Universities, the American Dental Association, and the Association of American Dental Colleges as well as existing national certification bodies, such as the various medical specialty boards and the National Board of Medical Examiners. Professional associations in the allied health fields would also be involved.

The time has come not only for serious consideration of uniform national standards but also for the removal of barriers to interstate mobility of all health professionals, with a view to encouraging more effective adjustment of supply to demand in the various states.

The Commission recommends the appointment of a National Health Manpower Commission to make a thorough study of changing patterns of education and utilization of health manpower, with particular reference to new types of allied health workers, of changing patterns of health care delivery, and of the feasibility of national licensing requirements for all health manpower.

ESTIMATED COST OF RECOMMENDED FEDERAL AID

The Commission's estimates of the cost of expanded federal financial support recommended in this report are as follows:

	Assuming continuation of four-year M.D.- and D.D.S.-candidate programs (in millions of constant dollars)	*Assuming that all schools shift to three-year programs by 1973–74 (in millions of constant dollars)*
1971–72	547.0	547.0
1972–73	635.8	635.8
1973–74	704.6	646.6
1974–75	770.9	623.9
1975–76	813.0	646.2
1976–77	857.5	671.7
1977–78	879.3	691.2
1978–79	908.1	719.3
1979–80	899.1	727.5

A breakdown of these costs is provided in Appendix B, Tables 3 and 4.

Total federal expenditures in 1969–70 for institutional support to medical and dental schools, scholarships and loans for medical and dental students, construction support for medical and dental schools, and Regional Medical Programs were approximately $275 million. Thus the added cost of the federal aid recommended by the Commission would be about $272 million in 1971–72.[4]

However, many of the Commission's recommendations would result in greater efficiency and, in the long run, a reduction in some types of federal support. Our cost estimates indicate substantial savings if all schools convert to three-year programs by 1973–74. Moreover, if this change should occur, there would be a case for discontinuation around 1980 of the policy of providing cost-of-education supplements to three-year schools *as if* they were four-year schools, since by that time the three-year programs would have been long established. In that case, there would be an additional saving in federal aid of about $80 million in 1971–72 dollars. In practice, some schools are likely to accelerate their programs by conducting summer sessions, as at the University of California, Irvine, and in that case there would be no cost reduction and no case for reducing the number of cost-of-education supplements to be received by the institution.

Moreover, widespread conversion to three-year programs would facilitate more rapid expansion of entrant classes than our projections indicate, with the result that some of the savings might be offset by additional expansion costs. The Commission believes that this possibility serves to emphasize the need for continuing studies of demand and supply of physicians and dentists throughout the 1970s to determine whether even more rapid expansion of entrant places than we have recommended would be desirable.

---

[4] The increase would actually be slightly larger than this comparison suggests, since the federal government treats the entire amount of a loan obtained in a given year as an expenditure, whereas our estimates include only the interest paid by the federal government when it borrows funds for the loan program as a cost, because the loan funds are revolving funds.

8. The Role of the States

Although the Commission is recommending substantially expanded federal support for medical and dental education, it considers a strong element of financial support from the states to be of critical importance to the continued development and expansion of institutions providing education for physicians and dentists. The federal financial support which we have recommended will not by any means cover the full operational costs of medical and dental education, nor will it cover full construction or start-up costs. Moreover, the states have a crucial role to play in the support of house officer education and educational programs for allied health manpower.

Since the majority of students undertaking residency training remain to practice in the states where they received their training, as indicated above, it is decidedly in the interest of states to contribute to the construction and development of institutions where residents are to be trained, including university health science centers and area health education centers. Furthermore, medical residents will not be attracted to states in which their compensation will be low. Thus it is in the interest of the states to make certain that residents are adequately compensated, to the extent that their compensation is not fully covered by charges for patient care, including payments through insurance and public programs such as Medicare and Medicaid. By the time students graduate from medical or dental school, they are likely to be heavily in debt and anxious to avoid incurring additional indebtedness during their postgraduate education.

In the development and expansion of programs for the education of allied health workers, the states must be expected to play the major role. Increasingly education in these rapidly expanding and proliferating occupations is being provided in comprehensive colleges and community colleges. Although these institutions and their students would benefit greatly from the expanded federal aid which the Commission has recommended in *Quality and Equality: Revised Recommendations, New Levels of Federal Responsibility for Higher Education,* we believe that the states should provide a substantial proportion of the financing of education in these colleges. Allied health workers, like house officers, tend to remain in the states where they were educated. Thus investment in their education provides a clearly demonstrable social return to the states.

In addition, the Commission believes that the states should provide financial support for private institutions involved in the education of health manpower. As indicated above, most of the medical schools that are encountering severe financial problems are private institutions. A number of them are parts of large urban universities which find that they cannot raise tuition sufficiently to meet rising costs.[1] Policies and criteria for state support for private institutions will be recommended in the Commission's forthcoming report *The Capitol and the Campus.*

The states should also play a very important role in the *planning* of health manpower education, in cooperation with the regional planning bodies and the universities. In some parts of the country, as suggested above, a regional conglomerate of several states may constitute a more rational planning entity than a state.

The variations in state financial support of medical and dental education are not only wide, but they also bear no rational relationship to differences in the financial capacity of the states (Map 3). This is strikingly revealed by a comparison of the ranking of the states in terms of expenditures on medical education per $100,000 of personal income with their ranking in per capita income (Table 5). On this basis the 10 states with the lowest expenditures in relation to per capita income were Delaware, Connecticut, Illinois, Massachusetts, Nevada, Rhode Island, New Jersey, Maryland, New Hampshire, and California. All these states were in the upper half of states in terms of per capita income.

On the other hand, the states that ranked high in expenditures in relation to per capita income were all in the lower half of states in terms of per capita income, and some of them were among the states with the very lowest incomes. They were Arkansas, Ken-

---

[1] A study being conducted for the Commission by Dr. Earl F. Cheit will provide detailed information on the adjustments being made by a number of institutions in financial difficulties, including the discontinuation of some of their professional education programs.

MAP 3 State expenditures for regular operating programs of medical schools per $100,000 personal income

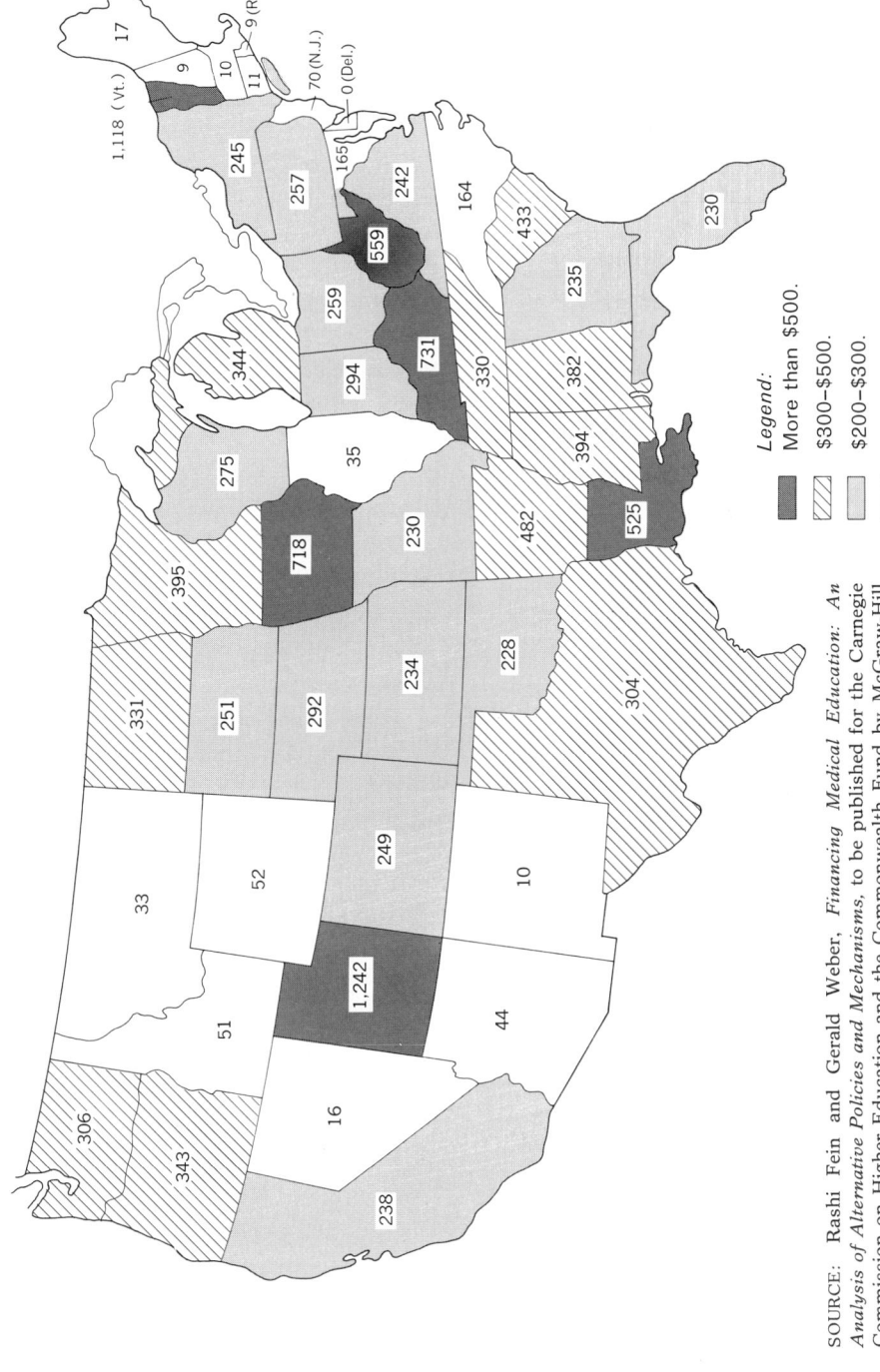

Legend:
More than $500.
$300–$500.
$200–$300.
Less than $200.

SOURCE: Rashi Fein and Gerald Weber, *Financing Medical Education: An Analysis of Alternative Policies and Mechanisms*, to be published for the Carnegie Commission on Higher Education and the Commonwealth Fund by McGraw-Hill Book Company, 1970.

TABLE 5
Ranking of states in expenditures for regular operating programs of medical schools per $100,000 personal income, compared with their ranking in per capita income, 1966*

State	Ranking in expenditures (1)	Ranking in per capita income (2)	Difference (2) − (1)
Utah	1	32	+31
Vermont	2	27	+25
Kentucky	3	42	+39
Iowa	4	18	+14
West Virginia	5	44	+39
Louisiana	6	40	+34
Arkansas	7	47	+40
South Carolina	8	46	+38
Minnesota	9	20	+11
Mississippi	10	48	+38
Alabama	11	45	+34
Michigan	12	11	− 1
Oregon	13	16	+ 3
North Dakota	14	36	+22
Tennessee	15	43	+28
Washington	16	8	− 8
Texas	17	31	+14
Indiana	18	12	− 6
Nebraska	19	22	+ 3
Wisconsin	20	17	− 3
Ohio	21	13	− 8
Pennsylvania	22	15	− 7
South Dakota	23	37	+14
Colorado	24	19	− 5
New York	25	4	−21
Virginia	26	28	+ 2
California	27	5	−22
Georgia	28	38	+10
Kansas	29	23	− 6
Florida	30.5	29	− 1.5
Missouri	30.5	21	− 9.5
Oklahoma	32	33	+ 1
Maryland	33	10	−23
North Carolina	34	41	+ 7
New Jersey	35	6	−29

State	Ranking in expenditures (1)	Ranking in per capita income (2)	Difference (2) − (1)
Wyoming	36	25	−11
Idaho	37	34	− 3
Arizona	38	30	− 8
Illinois	39	3	−36
Montana	40	26	−14
Maine	41	35	− 6
Nevada	42	7	−35
Connecticut	43	1	−42
Massachusetts	44.5	9	−35.5
New Mexico	44.5	39	− 5.5
New Hampshire	46.5	24	−22.5
Rhode Island	46.5	14	−32.5
Delaware	48	2	−46

*Expenditure data are averages for the academic years 1965 and 1966. Per capita income data are for 1966.

SOURCE: Map 3 and *Statistical Abstract of the United States, 1967*, p. 327.

tucky, West Virginia, Mississippi, South Carolina, Alabama, Louisiana, Utah, Tennessee, and Vermont.

This odd and unusual set of relationships is partly, but not wholly, explained by the preponderance of private medical schools in the former group of states and of public medical schools in the latter. Of the 21 medical schools in the low-expenditure states in 1966, 14 were private, whereas, among the 14 medical schools in the high-expenditure states, 10 were public. Two of the low-expenditure states—Delaware and Nevada—had no medical school, although Nevada now has a developing school.

The ranking of the states in terms of medical and dental students (not including interns and residents) per 100,000 population differs appreciably from their ranking in terms of expenditures on medical education per $100,000 personal income, although some of the states which rank high by the former measure also rank high by the latter (Map 4).[2] The 10 leading states on the basis of the former

[2] Medical students include M.D. candidates, postgraduate students in the basic sciences in medical schools, clinical fellows, and students in other health fields in medical schools in terms of equivalency to medical students with respect to faculty teaching responsibilities (45, p. 1561). Dental students include D.D.S. candidates; students in dental hygienist, dental assistant, and laboratory technician programs; and postgraduate dental students (32, pp. 12–13, 25).

MAP 4 Medical and dental students (other than interns and residents) per 100,000 population, by state, 1968

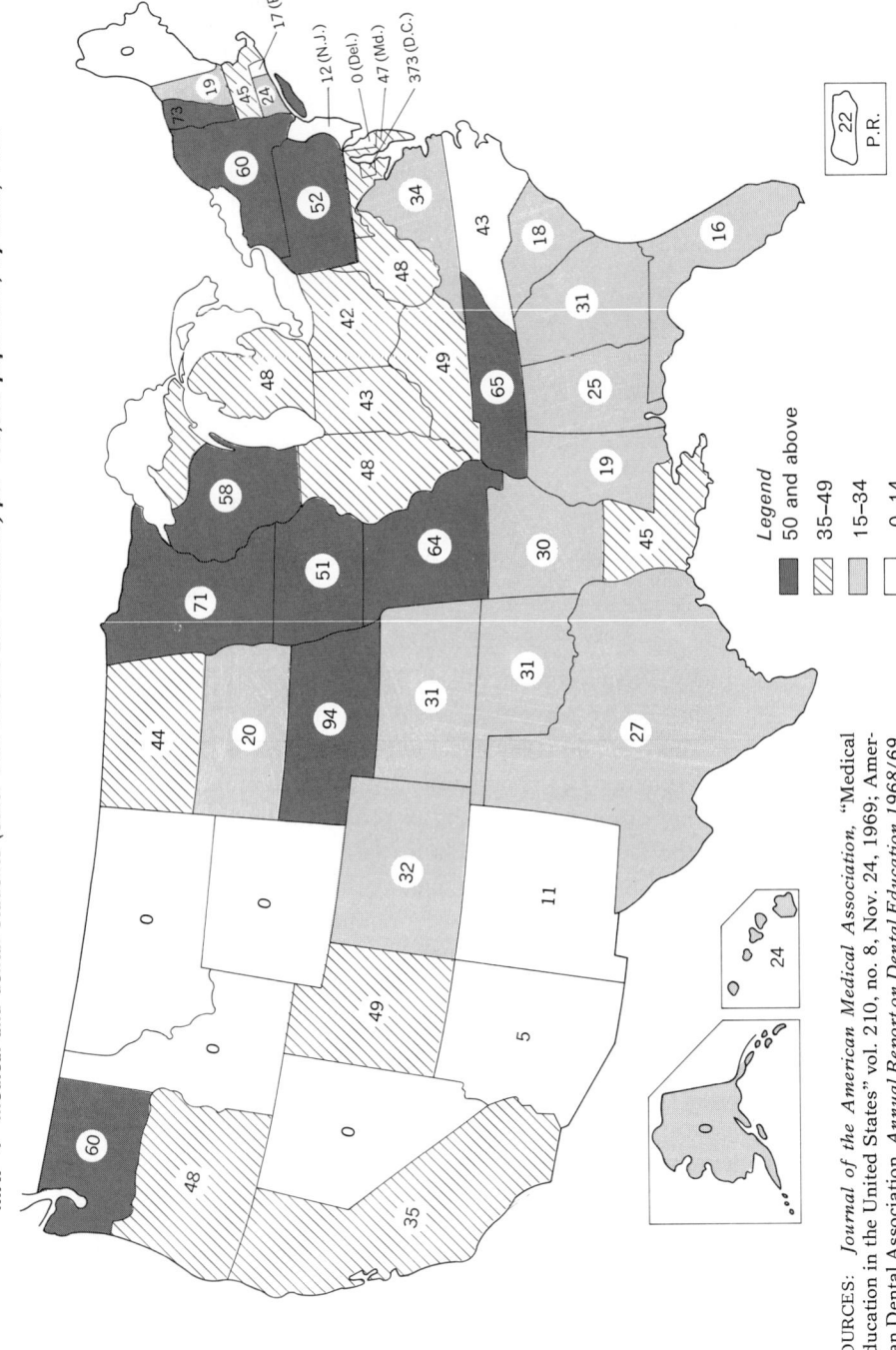

SOURCES: *Journal of the American Medical Association,* "Medical Education in the United States" vol. 210, no. 8, Nov. 24, 1969; American Dental Association, *Annual Report on Dental Education 1968/69,* part 1; *Statistical Abstract of the United States,* 1969, p. 12.

measure in 1968 were the District of Columbia (treated as a state for this purpose), Nebraska, Vermont, Tennessee, Missouri, New York, Washington, Wisconsin, Pennsylvania, and Iowa.

At the opposite end of the spectrum were the seven states without any medical or dental students—Alaska, Delaware, Idaho, Maine, Montana, Nevada (whose developing school had not yet admitted students), and Wyoming. Except in the case of Delaware, and Nevada, with its developing school, the Commission does not recommend new medical schools for these states because they lack cities or metropolitan areas with a population of at least 350,000. Instead, we are suggesting the development of area health education centers in these sparsely settled states.

One of the major functions of area health education centers, as previously suggested, would be the development of residency programs. There were seven states—Alaska, Idaho, Montana, Nevada, North and South Dakota, and Wyoming—that had no interns or residents in hospitals affiliated with medical schools in 1969 (Map 5). Other states that ranked very low in the number of interns and residents in affiliated hospitals per 100,000 population in 1969 were Maine, New Jersey, South Carolina, Arkansas, Indiana, Hawaii, Mississippi, West Virginia, Arizona, Alabama, and Iowa. Although some of these states had significant number of interns and residents in unaffiliated hospitals, most of them did not. The proportion of interns and residents in affiliated hospitals has been increasing rapidly, and, by 1968-69, 86 percent of all house officers who were United States medical graduates were in affiliated hospitals, while the proportion of foreign medical graduates in affiliated hospitals was somewhat smaller.

The states that lack interns and residents, or that have them in very small numbers, tend to be those with low per capita income. This is not, however, true of New Jersey, which ranked seventh in per capita income among the states in 1968.

Apart from the District of Columbia, which is unusually well endowed with medical schools in relation to its population, the states which had exceptionally large numbers of interns and residents in affiliated hospitals in relation to population were Minnesota, with its Mayo Clinic, and New York. Other states which ranked above the national average of 18 per 100,000 population were Vermont, Maryland, Massachusetts, Colorado, Connecticut, Rhode Island, Illinois, Pennsylvania, and Michigan—nearly all states with outstanding medical schools.

MAP 5 Interns and residents (M.D.'s) in hospitals affiliated with medical schools per 100,000 population, by state, 1969

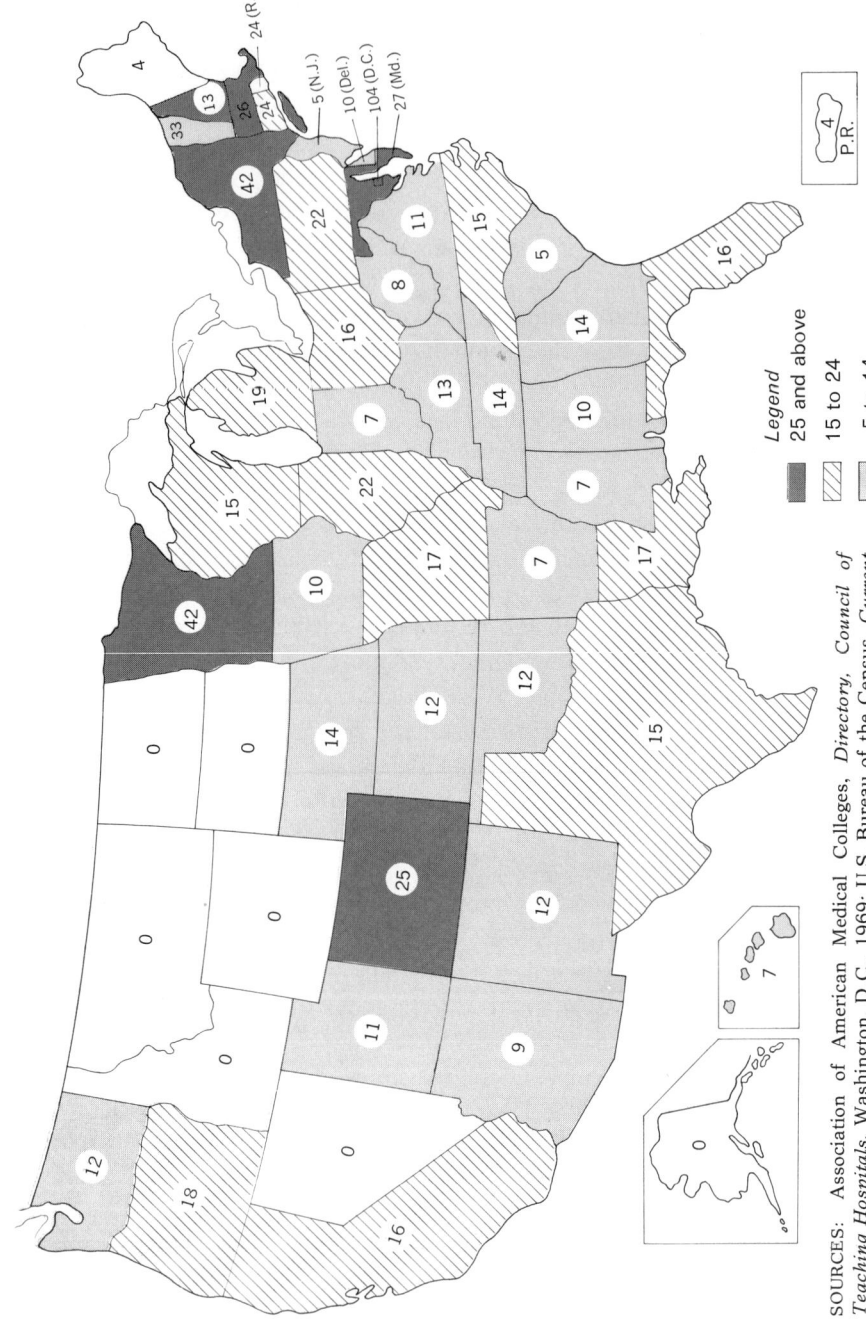

SOURCES: Association of American Medical Colleges, *Directory, Council of Teaching Hospitals*, Washington, D.C., 1969; U.S. Bureau of the Census, *Current Population Reports: Population Estimates and Projections*, ser. P-25, no. 436, Jan. 7, 1970.

The extremely uneven geographic distribution of interns and residents underscores the importance of the Commission's recommendation for the development of area health education centers, but in states with low per capita income special financial and nonfinancial incentives may also be required to attract residents to such centers and to induce them to remain in these states to practice later.

Our analysis of the geographic distribution of expenditures on medical education, of medical and dental students, and of interns and residents clearly indicates that a good many states have lagged seriously in support of medical and dental education. To the extent that these are states with low per capita income, this is understandable, but a number of the states with high per capita income have been seriously deficient in public support of medical and dental education. In some cases, as in Massachusetts, the deficiency is associated with the historical development of outstanding private institutions, but, as suggested above, many of the private institutions are now encountering serious financial problems and will require both federal and state support to maintain and expand their programs.

States with low expenditures should be expected to increase their contributions, particularly by supporting private medical schools, and the federal government, as noted above, should encourage them to do so as it negotiates levels of support.

Along with its recommendation for uniform tuition, the Commission also believes that medical and dental schools should be required to abolish state residency requirements and differential tuition for out-of-state students. Geographic considerations for admissions of students should not include preference for local residents; concern for a representative mixture from various regions of the United States and foreign countries should continue to be an important element of the educational experience.

The Commission recommends that states should continue to provide substantial financial support for medical and dental education and that states that have lagged in that past should plan for significant increases in expenditures for this purpose. The Commission recommends; also, that the states should provide financial support for medical and dental education in private institutions. In addition, the states should provide major financial support for house officer training and for the education of allied health personnel. The states, in cooperation with universities and with regional and local planning bodies, should also play a major role in the development of plans for the location of university health science centers, area health education centers, and comprehensive colleges and community colleges providing training for allied health personnel.

9. The Role of the Universities

Universities with affiliated health science centers should encourage these institutions to orient themselves toward assuming a central role in devising and supervising more coordinated and integrated health personnel education systems. They should also cooperate with other community bodies in the development of more effective systems of health care delivery. This will require major internal changes within the universities and their schools to enable them to increase greatly their public service role, develop new and more inclusive educational programs for health care personnel, and emphasize research on health delivery systems and medical sociology.

Among the responsibilities which they should undertake are:

1 To cooperate with other agencies in helping to develop more effective health care delivery systems in their communities and surrounding areas

2 To expand their medical and dental programs, to achieve acceleration and improved efficiency in these programs, and to introduce other curriculum reforms along the lines recommended in this report

3 To include medical economists, administration specialists, and behavioral scientists in their academic and service functions and to increase the educational emphasis in these fields as well as in preventive medicine and community health

4 To develop more effective integrated educational programs for the total health care team, including new specialties where needed, such as physician's associates and assistants, and to cooperate in the development of educational programs for allied health specialties conducted in comprehensive colleges and community colleges

5 To bring about a significant increase in continuing education programs for health care personnel in the area
6 To place greater emphasis on teaching as a rewarding scholarly activity for the faculty, especially in connection with salary and promotion policies
7 To undertake extensive research, in cooperation with appropriate university departments (economics, sociology, psychology, political science, etc.), on health care delivery systems

The university administration must, of course, play a major role in the development of plans for the expansion of university health science centers, working closely with regional and state planning agencies. In many cases, however, it is likely that the faculty and administration of the university health science centers will be oriented to research objectives to such an extent that they will not be prepared to expand the education and community planning roles of the centers in the manner envisaged in this report or to develop some of the new types of research recommended. Thus, it may be desirable in many universities to appoint a vice-president for health science affairs who will be concerned not only with plans for expansion but also with the changes in emphasis which the Commission envisages.

The university medical centers, moreover, are not organized administratively to undertake the broad roles that this report envisages for university health science centers. Without administrative reorganization, the result of any attempt to assume this expanded role might well be disastrous ineffectiveness. The Commission believes that universities should undertake careful study of this administrative problem and that in some cases the solution may well be a dual line of administration, with a dean in charge of academic programs and another administrator in charge of programs involving relations with other community agencies. In other cases, committees with specific functions may be more appropriate.

In their analyses of needed administrative changes, some of the very large universities may wish to consider the establishment of a separate advisory board for the university health science center and perhaps, in some cases, also for the teaching hospital, but the feasibility of such changes will vary among institutions.

Moreover, there is a need for much more careful integration of instruction in the biomedical sciences and in the social sciences between the health science centers and the campuses of the universities. To a large extent, this integration should be accomplished, whenever feasible, through joint appointments of faculty members.

The Commission recommends that university administrations appoint appropriate officers to develop plans for the expansion of university health science centers and for their transformation to perform the broad educational, research, and community service functions recommended in this report. University administrations should also be actively involved in the planning of area health education centers. To accomplish these objectives will often require administrative changes in the university and in the health science center as well. Careful integration of instruction in the biomedical sciences and social sciences between university health science centers and departments on major university campuses should be achieved.

10. The Role of the Comprehensive Colleges and Community Colleges

The rapid expansion of demand for workers in the allied health professions is creating an increasing need for curricula designed to prepare young people for these professions in both four-year comprehensive colleges and two-year public community colleges. Some of these institutions have responded to the need by expanding existing programs and introducing well-planned curricula designed to provide training for the many new technical specialties in the health field. Elsewhere the response has been limited. As the Commission's report *The Open-Door Colleges: Policies for Community Colleges* pointed out, some of the states have taken vigorous steps to stimulate the development of such systems; elsewhere there has been little or no development of community colleges. Implementation of the Commission's recommendations for federal aid to higher education is essential if development of comprehensive colleges and community colleges is to be stimulated in the laggard states.

Just as the university health science centers and area health education centers must become increasingly involved in cooperating with the comprehensive colleges and community colleges in planning such curricula, so these colleges should welcome advice from the centers in developing their training programs in the allied health professions.

The Allied Health Professions Personnel Training Act of 1966 has provided expanded federal support for education in these critically important health fields and has contributed significantly to the development and expansion of allied health programs in comprehensive and community colleges (56).

The Commission recommends that comprehensive colleges and community colleges develop and expand their curricula in the allied health professions where this has not been done and that they also seek and accept guidance from university health science centers and area health education centers in the planning and evaluation of these educational programs.

11. The Role of the Foundations

Some of the large private foundations have played an important role in providing financial support for medical education and research and in sponsoring studies of medical education. The Commission believes that the foundations should continue to give favorable consideration to proposals for this type of support and should also provide funds for research on health manpower and on problems in the delivery of health care. It is often more feasible for foundations to support studies or projects that are innovative or experimental than for government agencies to provide such support.

The Commission recommends that private foundations that have traditionally provided support for health manpower education and research should continue to do so and that foundations that have not provided such support in the past should consider expanding their programs to include it. The Commission also recommends that foundations expand their support for research on the delivery of health care.

12. Carnegie Commission Goals To Be Achieved by 1980

- Expansion of the functions of university health science centers so that they can play a central role in coordinating and guiding health manpower education and cooperating with other agencies in the development of improved health care delivery systems in their regions
- Development and expansion of programs for physician's and dentist's associates and assistants
- Acceleration of medical and dental education, thereby achieving greater efficiency
- Integration of the curriculum, including such changes as consolidation of instruction in the basic sciences on main university campuses, integration of preprofessional and professional education, and more carefully integrated and coordinated programs of postgraduate training
- Changes in medical and dental education so that they are more responsive to the expressed needs of students and more concerned with problems of delivery of health care
- A 50 percent increase in medical school entrant places
- Initiation of nine new university health science centers
- Positive policies to encourage the admission of women and members of minority groups to professional training in medicine and dentistry
- A 20 percent increase in dental school entrant places
- Development of approximately 126 area health education centers, affiliated with university health science centers

Appendix A: Joint Statements of the American Medical Association and the Association of American Medical Colleges, March 5, 1968, and April 16, 1968

MARCH 5, 1968

To meet national expectations for health services the enrollment of our nation's medical schools must be substantially increased. At a joint meeting held in Chicago on February 28, 1968, the representatives of the Board of Trustees of the American Medical Association and the Executive Council of the Association of American Medical Colleges emphasized the urgent and critical need for more physicians if national expectations for health services are to be realized.

National policy which would best meet this need and would be consistent with the American ideal of equal educational opportunity for all would provide such resources that every young person interested in and qualified for entry to the study of medicine would have this opportunity. Both Associations endorsed the position that all medical schools should now accept as a goal the expansion of their collective enrollments to a level that permits all qualified applicants to be admitted. As a nation, we should address the task of realizing this policy goal with a sense of great urgency.

In their endorsement of and call for broadening educational opportunity for the study of medicine, both Associations stressed that the length of time necessary to realize such a goal does not minimize the need to respond to today's critical shortage of physician manpower. In order to enable the nation's medical schools both to meet today's crisis and to attain the longer-range goal of unrestricted educational opportunity, those responsible for allocation of resources must recognize the magnitude of these tasks.

There are both immediate and long range steps which should be taken. The immediate steps are:

1 To increase the enrollment of existing medical schools. Considering the time required to create new schools and to provide a student with a medical education there is no alternative to this step in meeting our present emergency.

2 To foster curricular innovations and other changes in the educational programs which could shorten the time required for a medical education and minimize the costs. In view of the increasing quality of preprofessional education and the growing competence of entering medical students, it should be possible to reduce the length of medical education without sacrificing quality. Also, as the amount of clinical experience provided medical students increases, the duration of internship and residency training should be reassessed. The process of educating a physician embraces the entire curriculum from high school through residency training.

3 To meet the need for innovation in educational programs and to encourage diversity in the character and objectives of medical schools. The development of schools of quality where a primary mission is the preparation of able physicians for clinical practice as economically and rapidly as possible is to be encouraged. Such schools may have less emphasis upon fundamental biologic research than is appropriate for a number of other schools.

A longer range approach to the need for physicians is the development of new medical schools. This approach will not solve our immediate, urgent need for more physicians, but it is essential for meeting the national needs of 1980 and beyond. The contribution of such schools to the total capacity of the medical education systems is important. The advantages of the organization of as many such centers of medical education and development through the country as consistent with strong programs should be kept in mind.

To implement the measures enumerated above will require adequate financial support from governmental and various private sources for:

1 Construction of facilities to expand enrollment of existing schools and to create new schools.

2 Support of the operational costs of medical schools.
3 Stimulation and incentive for educational innovation and improvement.

To implement these measures will further require that each medical school and its university reexamine its objectives, its educational program, and its resources to determine how it can contribute most effectively to the national need for more physicians and what financial help it will need to make this contribution. Also required is understanding by the public, the private foundations, industry, local and state governments, and the national Congress groups which must provide the financial support which is necessary.

Initiative for development of new schools and expansion of established institutions should be locally determined. Only the governing bodies of schools with ongoing programs in medical education can decide to expand such programs. Institutions wishing to organize new medical schools must assume the responsibility for marshalling the necessary support. Both Associations are prepared to lend any assistance they can to such efforts.

APRIL 16, 1968

Rising public expectations for health services and determination to upgrade quickly the health care of large segments of the population have created unprecedented demands for physician manpower. The public's challenge to medical education to respond by producing the necessary health manpower is clearly understood and has been accepted by the medical profession. At a second joint meeting of members of the AMA Board of Trustees and the Executive Council of the AAMC, these groups again expressed their determination to mobilize the support necessary for the medical schools to expand enrollments to desirable levels.

A medical college is a complex, multi-purpose enterprise with important obligations to various individuals, groups, organizations, and to society. It is impossible for a medical college to operate at a high level and to discharge these obligations without effective funding, planning, coordination, and control. Appreciation of the complexity of function and financing is necessary for any understanding of the fiscal predicament in which academic medical centers now find themselves.

At this time AMA and AAMC urge that increased emphasis be given to support of the educational component of academic medical center activities with the intent that the production of physicians and other health personnel by such centers be assigned the highest possible priority. In their effort to mobilize support for medical education, AMA and AAMC leaders resolve to use all of their resources to achieve the desired results.

The problems of each academic medical center are unique to that institution. A blanket solution nationally designed and centrally imposed will not produce desired results. Rather, the interests and talents of governing boards, the magnitude and sources of assured support, the abilities and goals of faculties, the hopes and ambitions of students, and the influence of local, regional, and national attitudes must all go into determining in what fashion each academic medical center can make its optimal contribution.

A Increased Number of Graduates

    1 Increased Enrollment

Each medical school is examining carefully what it can do. In September, 1968, about 200 more students will enroll in the first year classes of all existing medical schools than in the fall of 1967. By 1969 another increment of over 400 is expected. Incentives should be devised to assist those schools which elect to expand enrollment with increased construction funds and operating budgets.

    2 More Medical Centers

In September, 1967, five new medical schools opened their doors, and in 1968 five others are expected to begin operation. Cities with a combination of population density, a strong undergraduate school, availability of adequate land, appropriate clinical facilities, and a reasonable source of financial support have been and should continue to be strongly encouraged when they seek to organize medical schools.

B Mobilization of Support

    1 From Local Sources

The AMA is asking its field staff to highlight the urgency of the manpower question before county and state medical societies. These societies will be asked to form committees to marshall a response at city, county, and state levels aimed at increased production of health manpower in both privately and publicly owned medical schools.

2 From Private Sources

Private sources—individuals, industries, and foundations—remain the largest contributors to the support of medical education. This fact must never be obscured by the prominence of federal and state tax support. Private support has allowed American medical education the flexibility which has made it strong. The AMA through its Education and Research Foundation and the AAMC in cooperation with the National Fund for Medical Education should join forces to convince industry and the foundations that it is in their vital interest to encourage diversity in the support of American medical education.

3 From the Federal Government

Federal support for the educational component of medical center activity should be further encouraged. The full sums of money authorized under existing legislation should be appropriated. Both AMA and AAMC have testified repeatedly and will continue to testify before both Senate and House committees during the coming year. Their testimony is virtually identical in request for support for medical education linked to increased enrollments. Passage of the Health Manpower Act of 1968, which provides for funding for construction, operation and educational innovation in medical centers, is being strongly advocated by both Associations.

C Other Specific Steps

In addition to the above-mentioned testimony before Congress for support of full appropriations for existing legislation, the call for passage of the Health Manpower Act of 1968, the development of local committees in state and county medical societies, and coordinated approaches to industry and other private sources, other measures are underway. Medical schools are (a) continuing to seek ways to enroll more students and to reduce dropout rates; (b) exploring methods for allowing entry into medical schools from many backgrounds, and at different levels; (c) organizing curricula which will permit progress through medical school at different rates; and (d) introducing measures to increase the educational effectiveness and productivity of medical schools. The modern medical curriculum, a continuum which includes college, medical school and the internship and residency years, is being examined with the objective of achieving optimal investment of the time of each student and faculty member.

The AMA and AAMC will continue to lend all of their support to a national program encompassing the features outlined in this statement.

Appendix B: Tables

TABLE 1 University health science centers and Carnegie Commission goals for new university health science centers and area health education centers by 1980, by state

State and city	Institution	Enrollment M.D. candidates	Total	Population
Alabama				
Birmingham	Medical College of Alabama	339	840	735,500*
Mobile	University health science center (developing)			383,200*
Dothan	Suggested area health education center			31,440†
Huntsville	Suggested area health education center			72,365†
Montgomery	Suggested area health education center (V.A. hospital).			134,393†
Alaska				
Anchorage	Suggested area health education center			44,237†
Fairbanks	Suggested area health education center			13,311†
Arizona				
Tucson	University of Arizona	63	79	212,892†
Phoenix	Recommended new university health science center			858,900*
Flagstaff	Suggested area health education center			18,214†
Arkansas				
Little Rock	University of Arkansas	395	723	318,800*
El Dorado	Suggested area health education center			25,292†
Fort Smith	Suggested area health education center			52,991†
California				
Davis	University of California	48	290	8,910†
Irvine	University of California	262	580	1,231,200*

Higher education and the nation's health 108

TABLE 1 University health science centers and Carnegie Commission goals for new university health science centers and area health education centers by 1980, by state   continued

		Enrollment		
State and city	Institution	M.D. candidates	Total	Population
Loma Linda	Loma Linda University	357	604	2,000†
Los Angeles	University of California	389	1,993	6,857,200*
	University of Southern California	289	1,474	6,857,200*
Palo Alto	Stanford University	327	927	959,200*
San Diego	University of California	47	230	1,198,100*
San Francisco	University of California	523	1,818	3,009,100*
Fresno	Recommended new university health science center (V.A. hospital)			415,700*
Bakersfield	Suggested area health education center			327,300*
Redding	Suggested area health education center			12,773†
Santa Rosa	Suggested area health education center			31,027†
Los Angeles	Five suggested area health education centers (V.A. hospital)			6,857,200*
San Bernardino	Suggested area health education center			1,085,900*
San Francisco-Oakland	Suggested area health education center (East Bay area)			3,009,100*
Colorado				
Denver	University of Colorado	360	982	1,089,800*
Grand Junction	Suggested area health education center			18,694†
Pueblo	Suggested area health education center			91,181†
Connecticut				
Hartford	University of Connecticut	32	56	793,400*
New Haven	Yale University	347	848	721,200*
Bridgeport	Suggested area health education center			772,700*
Waterbury	Suggested area health education center			107,130†
Delaware				
Wilmington	Recommended university health science center			481,000*
District of Columbia	Georgetown University	464	943	2,704,100*
	George Washington University	414	890	2,704,100*
	Howard University	393	899	2,704,100*

Appendix B: Tables

State and city	Institution	Enrollment M.D. candidates	Total	Population
Florida				
Gainesville	University of Florida	246	622	29,701†
Miami	University of Miami	332	982	1,114,000*
Tallahassee	Florida State University (developing)			48,237†
Tampa	University of South Florida (developing Fall 1971)			891,000*
Jacksonville	Recommended new university health science center			504,600*
Orlando	Suggested area health education center			383,900*
Georgia				
Atlanta	Emory University	293	1,018	1,288,500*
Augusta	Medical College of Georgia	393	615	70,626†
Columbus	Suggested area health education center			116,779†
Macon	Suggested area health education center			69,764†
Savannah	Suggested area health education center			149,245†
Hawaii				
Honolulu	University of Hawaii (2-year school)	59	191	619,500*
Hilo	Suggested area health education center			25,966†
Idaho				
Boise	Suggested area health education center (V.A. hospital)			34,481†
Pocatello	Suggested area health education center			28,534†
Illinois				
Chicago	Chicago Medical School	294	413	6,770,700*
	University of Chicago	289	939	6,770,700*
	University of Illinois	793	1,490	6,770,700*
	Chicago College of Osteopathy	301		6,770,700*
	Northwestern University	547	1,546	6,770,700*
	Loyola-Stritch School of Medicine	383	608	6,770,700*
	Rush Medical College (developing)			6,770,700*

TABLE 1 University health science centers and Carnegie Commission goals for new university health science centers and area health education centers by 1980, by state continued

State and city	Institution	Enrollment M.D. candidates	Total	Population
Carbondale-Springfield	University of Southern Illinois (developing)			97,941†
Peoria	University of Illinois (developing)			103,162†
Rockford	University of Illinois (developing)			126,706†
Champaign-Urbana	Suggested area health education center			76,877†
East St. Louis	Suggested area health education center			81,712†
Indiana				
Indianapolis	Indiana University	857	1,857	1,041,600*
Evansville	Suggested area health education center			141,543†
Fort Wayne	Suggested area health education center (V.A. hospital)			161,776†
Gary	Suggested area health education center			602,800*
South Bend	Suggested area health education center			271,400*
Terre Haute	Suggested area health education center			72,500†
Iowa				
Des Moines	College of Osteopathic Medicine and Surgery	348		208,982†
Iowa City	University of Iowa	494	1,311	33,443†
Davenport	Suggested area health education center			358,100*
Sioux City	Suggested area health education center			89,159†
Waterloo	Suggested area health education center			71,755†
Kansas				
Kansas City	University of Kansas	483	932	1,214,400*
Wichita	Recommended new university health science center	395	600	395,600*
Dodge City	Suggested area health education center			13,520†
Salina	Suggested area health education center			43,202†
Topeka	Suggested area health education center (V.A. hospital)			119,484†
Kentucky				
Lexington	University of Kentucky	300	674	62,810†
Louisville	University of Louisville	367	761	795,000*

Appendix B: Tables 111

State and city	Institution	Enrollment M.D. candidates	Total	Population
Ashland	Suggested area health education center			31,283†
Paducah	Suggested area health education center			34,479†
Louisiana				
New Orleans	Louisiana State University	510	830	1,059,100*
	Tulane University	506	1,015	1,059,100*
Shreveport	Louisiana State University, Shreveport School of Medicine (developing Fall 1969)			288,300*
Lake Charles	Suggested area health education center			63,392†
Maine				
Bangor	Suggested area health education center			38,912†
Presque Isle	Suggested area health education center			12,886†
Portland	Suggested area health education center			72,566†
Maryland				
Baltimore	Johns Hopkins University	373	1,046	1,990,000*
	University of Maryland	521	941	1,990,000*
Cumberland	Suggested area health education center			33,415*
Hagerstown	Suggested area health education center			36,660†
Massachusetts				
Boston	Boston University	306	880	3,249,800*
	Harvard Medical School	577	577§	3,249,800*
	Tufts University	458	1,044	3,249,800*
Worcester	University of Massachusetts School of Medicine (developing Fall 1970)			618,800*
Springfield	Recommended new university health science center			557,100*
Pittsfield	Suggested area health education center			57,879†
Michigan				
Ann Arbor	University of Michigan	807	2,601	67,340†
Detroit	Wayne State University	531	1,161	4,113,600*
East Lansing	Michigan State University	78	462	353,500*

TABLE 1 University health science centers and Carnegie Commission goals for new university health science centers and area health education centers by 1980, by state   continued

		Enrollment		
State and city	Institution	M.D. candidates	Total	Population
Pontiac	Michigan College of Osteopathic Medicine	20		82,233†
Detroit	Two suggested area health education centers			4,113,600*
Flint	Suggested area health education center			476,800*
Grand Rapids	Suggested area health education center			514,300*
Kalamazoo	Suggested area health education center			82,089†
Saginaw	Suggested area health education center (V.A. hospital)			98,265†
Minnesota				
Minneapolis	University of Minnesota	685	2,281	1,636,200*
Duluth-Superior	Recommended new university health science center			272,600*
Rochester	Mayo Clinic—existing area health education center			40,663†
St. Cloud	Suggested area health education center			33,815†
Mississippi				
Jackson	University of Mississippi	319	587	144,422†
Biloxi	Suggested area health education center (V.A. hospital)			44,053†
Greenville	Suggested area health education center			41,502†
Tupelo	Suggested area health education center			17,221†
Missouri				
Columbia	University of Missouri	358	1,079	36,650†
Kansas City	University of Missouri, Kansas City School of Medicine (developing Fall 1971)	0	0	1,214,400*
	Kansas City College of Osteopathy and Surgery	446		1,214,400*
Kirksville	Kirksville College of Osteopathy and Surgery	421		13,123†
St. Louis	St. Louis University	461	781	2,311,400*
	Washington University	359	871	2,311,400*
Springfield	Suggested area health education center			95,865†

Appendix B: Tables **113**

State and city	Institution	Enrollment M.D. candidates	Total	Population
Montana				
Billings	Suggested area health education center			52,851†
Butte	Suggested area health education center			27,877†
Miles City	Suggested area health education center (V.A. hospital)			9,665†
Nebraska				
Omaha	Creighton University	302	423	514,600*
	University of Nebraska	365	602	514,600*
Grand Island	Suggested area health education center (V.A. hospital)			25,742†
Lincoln	Suggested area health education center (V.A. hospital)			128,521†
North Platte	Suggested area health education center			17,184†
Nevada				
Reno	University of Nevada (developing Fall 1971) (V.A. hospital)			51,470†
Las Vegas	Suggested area health education center			64,405†
New Hampshire				
Hanover	Dartmouth Medical School (2-year school)	100	224	5,649†
Berlin	Suggested area health education center			17,821†
Manchester	Suggested area health education center			88,282†
New Jersey				
Jersey City	New Jersey College of Medicine and Dentistry	306	536	620,000*
New Brunswick	Rutgers Medical School (2-year school)	30	61	40,139†
Newark	New Jersey College of Medicine (campus under construction)			1,888,500*
Atlantic City	Suggested area health education center			59,544†
Camden	Suggested area health education center			117,159†
Patterson-Clifton-Passaic	Suggested area health education center			1,341,000*
Trenton	Suggested area health education center			114,167†

TABLE 1 University health science centers and Carnegie Commission goals for new university health science centers and area health education centers by 1980, by state continued

State and city	Institution	Enrollment M.D. candidates	Enrollment Total	Population
New Mexico				
Albuquerque	University of New Mexico School of Medicine	97	202	201,189†
Gallup	Suggested area health education center			14,089†
Roswell	Suggested area health education center			39,593†
New York				
Albany	Albany Medical College	284	997	710,200*
Brooklyn	State University of New York	770	1,471	11,555,900*
Buffalo	State University of New York	407	1,355	1,331,600*
New York City	Cornell University Medical College	353	826	11,555,900*
	Albert Einstein College of Medicine	402	1,204	11,555,900*
	Columbia University	499	1,612	11,555,900*
	Mt. Sinai School of Medicine	59	2,003	11,555,900*
	New York Medical College	495	944	11,555,900*
	New York University	514	1,209	11,555,900*
Rochester	University of Rochester	308	809	838,900*
Syracuse	State University of New York	399	786	619,100*
Stony Brook	State University of New York (developing Fall 1971)	0	0	3,548†
Cooperstown	Mary I. Bassett Hospital—existing area health education center			2,553†
Binghamton	Suggested area health education center			301,100*
New York City	Suggested area health education center			11,555,900*
Utica	Suggested area health education center			349,500*
North Carolina				
Chapel Hill	University of North Carolina	287	1,080	12,573†
Durham	Duke University	333	1,023	78,302†
Winston-Salem	Bowman-Gray School of Medicine	226	437	582,000*
Greenville	East Carolina University (developing)			22,860†
Asheville	Suggested area health education center			60,192†
Charlotte	Suggested area health education center			378,000*
Wilmington	Suggested area health education center			44,013†

		Enrollment		
State and city	Institution	M.D. candidates	Total	Population
North Dakota				
Grand Forks	University of North Dakota (2-year school)	98	276	34,451†
Fargo	Suggested area health education center (V.A. hospital)			46,662†
Minot	Suggested area health education center			30,604†
Ohio				
Cincinnati	University of Cincinnati	407	882	1,361,000*
Cleveland	Case Western Reserve University	374	1,391	2,050,100*
Columbus	Ohio State University	611	2,262	859,600*
Toledo	Medical College of Ohio (developing Fall 1969)	0	0	670,700*
Akron	Suggested area health education center			660,000*
Dayton	Suggested area health education center			820,400*
Lima	Suggested area health education center			51,037†
Mansfield	Suggested area health education center			47,325†
Youngstown-Warren	Suggested area health education center			525,400*
Oklahoma				
Oklahoma City	University of Oklahoma	418	997	597,900*
Tulsa	Recommended new university health science center			451,400*
Enid	Suggested area health education center			38,859†
Lawton	Suggested area health education center			61,697†
Oregon				
Portland	University of Oregon	351	846	933,300*
Eugene	Suggested area health education center			50,977†
Medford	Suggested area health education center			24,425†
Pennsylvania				
Hershey	Pennsylvania State University	88	104	6,851†
Philadelphia	Hahnemann Medical College	432	731	4,774,400*
	Jefferson Medical College	717	1,093	4,774,400*

TABLE 1 University health science centers and Carnegie Commission goals for new university health science centers and area health education centers by 1980, by state   continued

		Enrollment		
State and city	Institution	M.D. candidates	Total	Population
	Temple University	552	887	4,774,400*
	University of Pennsylvania	520	1,380	4,774,400*
	Woman's Medical College	237	342	4,774,400*
	Philadelphia College of Osteopathic Medicine	461		4,774,400*
Pittsburgh	University of Pittsburgh	388	924	2,386,100*
Allentown-Bethlehem-Easton	Suggested area health education center			525,500*
Altoona	Suggested area health education center (V.A. hospital)			69,407†
Erie	Suggested area health education center (V.A. hospital)			138,440†
Reading	Suggested area health education center			290,600*
Pittsburgh	Suggested area health education center			2,386,100*
Scranton-Wilkes-Barre-Hazleton	Suggested area health education center			579,000‡
York	Suggested area health education center			311,900*
Puerto Rico				
San Juan	University of Puerto Rico	268	584	225,000†
Mayaguez	Suggested area health education center			83,850†
Ponce	Suggested area health education center			99,000†
Rhode Island				
Providence	Brown University (2-year school)	20	313	749,100*
South Carolina				
Charleston	Medical College of South Carolina	326	599	69,925†
Columbia	Suggested area health education center (V.A. hospital)			97,433†
Greenville	Suggested area health education center			66,188†
South Dakota				
Vermillion	University of South Dakota (2-year school)	86	132	6,102†

		Enrollment		
State and city	Institution	M.D. candidates	Total	Population
Rapid City	Suggested area health education center			42,399†
Sioux Falls	Suggested area health education center			65,466†
Tennessee				
Memphis	University of Tennessee	738	1,362	760,500*
Nashville	Meharry Medical College	278	379	531,100*
	Vanderbilt University	227	709	531,100*
Chattanooga	Suggested area health education center			299,000*
Knoxville	Suggested area health education center			393,500*
Texas				
Dallas	University of Texas Southwestern	411	1,068	1,404,800*
Galveston	University of Texas Medical Branch	606	945	67,175†
Houston	Baylor University	351	857	1,787,600*
	University of Texas Medical School (developing Fall 1971)			1,787,600*
San Antonio	University of Texas Medical School	105	265	834,000*
Lubbock	Texas Technological University (developing)			128,691†
Amarillo	Suggested area health education center (V.A. hospital)			137,969†
Beaumont	Suggested area health education center			315,500*
Corpus Christi	Suggested area health education center			292,400*
El Paso	Suggested area health education center			348,300*
Fort Worth	Suggested area health education center			657,700*
Odessa	Suggested area health education center			80,338†
Utah				
Salt Lake City	University of Utah	259	661	189,454†
Cedar City	Suggested area health education center			7,543†
Vermont				
Burlington	University of Vermont	232	462	35,531†
Rutland	Suggested area health education center			18,305†

TABLE 1 University health science centers and Carnegie Commission goals for new university health science centers and area health education centers by 1980, by state — continued

State and city	Institution	Enrollment M.D. candidates	Total	Population
Virginia				
Charlottesville	University of Virginia	319	697	29,427†
Richmond	Medical College of Virginia	451	1,037	508,500*
Norfolk-Portsmouth	Recommended new university health science center (V.A. hospital nearby at Hampton)			646,400*
Roanoke	Suggested area health education center			97,110†
Washington				
Seattle	University of Washington	334	1,940	1,261,600*
Spokane	Suggested area health education center (V.A. hospital)			266,300*
Walla Walla	Suggested area health education center			24,536†
Yakima	Suggested area health education center			43,284†
West Virginia				
Morgantown	West Virginia University	250	667	22,487†

*Estimated population of Standard Metropolitan Statistical Areas, 1967, from U.S. Bureau of the Census, *Current Population Reports: Population Estimates,* ser. P-25, no. 411, Washington, D.C., 1968.

†Population of urban place, from *U.S. Census of Population, 1960.*

‡1967 population of Wilkes-Barre-Hazelton, plus 1960 population of Lackawanna County, of which Scranton is the county seat.

§ Interns, residents, and other postdoctoral students were not reported.

Appendix B: Tables **119**

State and city	Institution	Enrollment M.D. candidates	Total	Population
Charleston	Suggested area health education center			87,796†
Parkersburg	Suggested area health education center			44,797†
Wisconsin				
Madison	University of Wisconsin	403	1,307	126,706†
Milwaukee	Marquette University	412	1,001	1,342,400*
Eau Claire	Suggested area health education center			37,987†
Green Bay	Suggested area health education center			62,888†
Wausau	Suggested area health education center			31,943†
Wyoming				
Casper	Suggested area health education center			38,930†
Cheyenne	Suggested area health education center (V.A. hospital)			43,505†
TOTAL ENROLLMENT		35,833	89,195	

SOURCE: American Medical Association: *Medical Education in the United States, 1968–69,* Chicago, 1969, pp. 1467 and 1560–1561. Identification of locations of recommended university health science centers and area health education centers is based on analyses by the Carnegie Commission staff. Enrollment data are for 1968–69, and developing medical schools with no enrollment figures had not admitted any students by that time.

**TABLE 2
Enrollment in dental schools, United States, fall, 1968**

State	Institution	Total enrollment, 1968*
Alabama	University of Alabama	258
California	University of the Pacific	304
	University of California	364
	University of California at Los Angeles	295
	University of Southern California	518
	Loma Linda University	334
Connecticut	University of Connecticut	17
District of Columbia	Georgetown University	428
	Howard University	353
Georgia	Emory University	318
Illinois	Loyola University of Chicago	513
	Northwestern University	417
	University of Illinois	458
Indiana	Indiana University	567
Iowa	University of Iowa	340
Kentucky	University of Kentucky	237
	University of Louisville	261
Louisiana	Louisiana State University	30
	Loyola University, New Orleans	248
Maryland	University of Maryland	402
Massachusetts	Harvard University	76
	Tufts University	481
Michigan	University of Detroit	448
	University of Michigan	552
Minnesota	University of Minnesota	343
Missouri	Saint Louis University	192
	University of Missouri at Kansas City	582
	Washington University	217

*Includes D.D.S. candidates and students in dental hygienist, dental assistant, and laboratory tecnhician programs and in postgraduate dental studies.

State	Institution	Total enrollment, 1968*
Nebraska	Creighton University	192
	University of Nebraska	263
New Jersey	Fairleigh Dickinson University	299
	New Jersey College of Dentistry	181
New York	Columbia University	250
	New York University	908
	State University of New York at Buffalo	319
North Carolina	University of North Carolina	291
Ohio	Ohio State University	805
	Case Western Reserve University	261
Oregon	University of Oregon	378
Pennsylvania	Temple University	654
	University of Pennsylvania	693
	University of Pittsburgh	573
South Carolina	Medical College of South Carolina	47
Tennessee	Meharry Medical College	151
	University of Tennessee	484
Texas	Baylor University	512
	University of Texas	528
Virginia	Medical College of Virginia	319
Washington	University of Washington	420
West Virginia	West Virginia University	297
Wisconsin	Marquette University	641
Puerto Rico	University of Puerto Rico	174
TOTAL		19,193

SOURCE: American Dental Association, *Annual Report on Dental Education, 1968-69,* part 1, Chicago, 1969.

TABLE 3
Estimated cost of federal aid for medical and dental education,* assuming continuation of four-year program, 1971–72 to 1979–80 (in millions of constant dollars)

Year	Student grants	Student loans	Cost-of-instruction supplements	Construction grants
1971–72	64.6	2.0	329.8	75.6
1972–73	69.8	4.0	369.7	117.3†
1973–74	75.6	6.2	411.1	136.7
1974–75	82.4	9.2	450.2	154.1
1975–76	87.1	11.9	486.0	153.0
1976–77	91.7	14.7	524.1	152.0
1977–78	96.1	17.5	564.0	141.7
1978–79	100.1	21.5	598.4	128.1
1979–80	103.1	23.2	618.7	94.1

*Does not include federal aid for biomedical research, which was included in the estimated cost of federal aid recommendations in Quality and Equality: Revised Recommendations, New Levels of Federal Responsibility for Higher Education.
†Includes $10 million a year for expansion of area health education centers from 1972–73 on.
SOURCE: Carnegie Commission staff.

TABLE 4
Estimated cost of federal aid for medical and dental education* assuming that all schools shift to three-year programs by 1973–74, 1971–72 to 1979–80 (in millions of constant dollars)

Year	Student grants	Student loans	Cost-of-instruction supplements	Construction grants
1971–72	64.6	2.0	329.8	75.6
1972–73	69.8	4.0	369.7	117.3†
1973–74	73.9	6.1	406.1	85.5
1974–75	75.1	8.2	432.7	32.9
1975–76	73.7	10.3	454.3	32.9
1976–77	71.4	12.2	478.5	34.6
1977–78	74.8	14.2	505.8	36.4
1978–79	77.6	16.2	529.1	36.4
1979–80	79.8	18.3	533.0	36.4

*Does not include federal aid for biomedical research, which was included in the estimated cost of federal aid recommendations in Quality and Equality: New Levels of Federal Responsibility for Higher Education.
†Includes $10 million a year for expansion of area health education centers from 1972–73 on.
SOURCE: Carnegie Commission staff.

Start-up grants	Regional planning	Continuing education	Total
15.0	50.0	10.0	547.0
15.0	50.0	10.0	635.8
15.0	50.0	10.0	704.6
15.0	50.0	10.0	770.9
15.0	50.0	10.0	813.0
15.0	50.0	10.0	857.5
	50.0	10.0	879.3
	50.0	10.0	908.1
	50.0	10.0	899.1

Start-up grants	Regional planning	Continuing education	Total
15.0	50.0	10.0	547.0
15.0	50.0	10.0	635.8
15.0	50.0	10.0	646.6
15.0	50.0	10.0	623.9
15.0	50.0	10.0	646.2
15.0	50.0	10.0	671.7
	50.0	10.0	691.2
	50.0	10.0	719.3
	50.0	10.0	727.5

References

1. Rutstein, D. D.: *The Coming Revolution in Medicine,* The MIT Press, Cambridge, Mass., and London, 1967.
2. *Statistical Abstract of the United States, 1969.*
3. United Nations: *Population and Vital Statistics Report,* ser. A, vol. 21, no. 1, Jan. 1, 1969, and no. 2, April 1, 1969.
4. U.S. Social Security Administration: *Social Security Programs throughout the World,* Washington, D.C., 1967.
5. U.S. Public Health Service: *Total Loss of Teeth in Adults,* Washington, D.C., 1967.
6. U.S. Public Health Service: *Dental Visits: Time Interval Since Last Visit, U.S.,* July 1963 and June 1964, Washington, D.C., 1966.
7. *The New York Times,* June 11, 1970.
8. "Country's No. 1 Health Problem: Interview with Top Presidential Adviser," *U.S. News and World Report,* February 23, 1970, pp. 68–73.
9. Cordtz, D.: "Change Begins in the Doctor's Office," *Fortune,* pp. 84–89, 130–134, January 1970.
10. Tucker, M.: "Utilization and Price Analysis: Prospects for Avoiding Higher Program Costs in Health Care," *American Journal of Public Health,* 59: 1226–1242 (July 1969).
11. *Report of the National Advisory Commission on Health Manpower,* 2 vols., Washington, D.C., 1967.
12. Skolnik, A. M., and S. R. Dales: "Social Welfare Expenditures, 1968–69," *Social Security Bulletin,* 32:3–18 (December 1969).
13. Reed, L. S.: "Private Health Insurance, 1968: Enrollment, Coverage, and Financial Experience," *Social Security Bulletin,* 32:19–35 (December 1969).
14. Rice, D. P., and B. S. Cooper: "National Health Expenditures, 1929–68," *Social Security Bulletin,* 33:3–20 (January 1970).

15 "National Commission for the Study of Nursing and Nursing Education: Summary Report and Recommendations," *American Journal of Nursing,* **70**:279–294 (February 1970).

16 Flexner, A.: *Medical Education in the United States and Canada,* A report to The Carnegie Foundation for the Advancement of Teaching; Bulletin no. 4, D. B. Updike, The Merrymount Press, Boston, 1910.

17 U.S. Public Health Service: *Health Resources Statistics,* 1968, Washington, D.C., 1968.

18 Lopate, Carol: *Women in Medicine,* The Johns Hopkins Press, Baltimore, 1968.

19 *Needed: Female Applicants, Target: Dental Education,* American Association of Dental Schools, vol. 2, no. 1, June 1967.

20 Powers, L., R. D. Parmelle, and H. Wiesenfelder: "Practice Patterns of Women and Men Physicians," *Journal of Medical Education,* **44**:481–491 (June 1969).

21 Haynes, M. A.: "Distribution of Black Physicians in the United States, 1967," *Journal of the American Medical Association,* **210**:93–95 (October 6, 1969).

22 *Report of the Association of American Medical Colleges Task Force to the Inter-Association Committee on Expanding Educational Opportunities in Medicine for Blacks and Other Minority Students,* April 22, 1970.

23 Crowley, A. E., and H. C. Nicholson: "Negro Enrollment in Medical Schools," *Journal of the American Medical Association,* **210**:96–100 (October 6, 1969).

24 Applewhite, H. L.: "The Vanishing Negro Dentist," *Quarterly of the National Dental Association,* **27**:78–79 (April 1969).

25 Fein, R., and G. Weber: *The Financing of Medical Education,* to be published by the McGraw-Hill Book Company for the Carnegie Commission on Higher Education, 1970.

26 Garfield, S. R.: "The Delivery of Medical Care," *Scientific American,* **222**: 15–23 (April 1970).

27 Fein, R.: *The Doctor Shortage,* The Brookings Institution, Washington, D.C., 1967.

28 Folger, J. K., H. S. Astin, and A. E. Bayer: *Human Resources and Higher Education,* Russell Sage Foundation, New York, 1970.

29 Blumberg, M. S.: *Medicine,* unpublished paper, University of California, 1969.

30 Blumberg, M. S.: *Dentistry and Related Occupations,* unpublished paper, University of California, 1969.

31 "Number of Dental Graduates Required Annually to 1985," *Journal of the American Dental Association*, 71:694–695 (September 1965).

32 **American Dental Association:** *Annual Report on Dental Education, 1968–69,* Chicago, 1969.

33 Millis, J. S.: "Which Way Dental Education?" *Journal of the American College of Dentists*, 35:5–14 (January 1968).

34 Roder, D. M.: "The New Zealand Dental Nurse: Observations on the Scene and in the Literature," *Journal of the American College of Dentists*, 35:257–264 (July 1968).

35 Estes, E. H., Jr., and D. R. Howard: "Potential for New Classes of Personnel: Experiences of the Duke Physician's Assistant Program," *Journal of Medical Education*, 45:149–155 (March 1970).

36 Silver, H. K., and J. A. Hecker: "The Pediatric Nurse Practitioner and the Child Health Associate: New Types of Health Professionals," *Journal of Medical Education*, 45:171–176 (March 1970).

37 **Sanazaro, P. J.:** *The R&D Approach to Health Manpower in the 1970's,* paper presented at the Conference on Physician Support Personnel, American Medical Association, Chicago, March 19, 1970.

38 **Fenderson, D.A.:** *Manpower for a System of Health Care,* paper presented at the Rural Health Conference, Brookings, South Dakota, May 2, 1970.

39 **The American Assembly, Columbia University:** *The Health of Americans,* report of the Thirty-seventh American Assembly, Arden House, Harriman, New York, April 23–26, 1970.

40 Field, J.: "Medical Education in the United States: Late Nineteenth and Twentieth Centuries," in C. D. O'Malley (ed.), *The History of Medical Education,* University of California Press, Los Angeles, 1970, pp. 501–530.

41 **University of Michigan:** *Integrated Flexible Medical-Premedical Curriculum,* October 21, 1969.

42 **Harvard Medical School:** *Memorandum of Dean Robert Ebert to Members of the Faculty of Medicine,* March 4, 1970.

43 **University of Illinois:** *A Plan for the Reorganization and Expansion of the College of Medicine,* November 4, 1969.

44 **Association of American Medical Colleges:** *Medical School Admission Requirements, U.S.A. and Canada, 1969–70,* Washington, D.C., 1969.

45 **American Medical Association:** *Medical Education in the United States, 1968–69,* Chicago, 1969.

46 Rogers, D. E.: "A Dean's List of Proposals," *Medical Opinion and Review,* 5:24–33 (October 1969).

47 *The Graduate Education of Physicians,* The report of the Citizens Commission on Graduate Medical Education (John S. Millis, chairman), commissioned by the American Medical Association, Chicago, 1967.

48 *Bulletin of the Association of American Medical Colleges,* 5:1, 6–7 (June 13, 1970)

49 *Bulletin of the Association of American Medical Colleges,* 5:1–8 (June 29, 1970).

50 *Higher Education and National Affairs,* 19:8–12 (June 17, 1970).

51 *Educational Opportunity Bank,* a report of the Panel on Educational Innovation to the U.S. Commissioner of Education, the Director of the National Science Foundation, and the Special Assistant to the President for Science and Technology, Government Printing Office, Washington, D.C., 1967.

52 Shell, K.: "A New Approach to the Financing of Medical Education," *Harvard Medical Alumni Bulletin,* 43:2–4 (Winter, 1969).

53 Bain, H.: "RMP: ℞ for Home Rule in Health Care," *SDC Magazine,* 12:3–12 (September 1969).

54 **National Science Foundation, National Register of Scientific and Technical Personnel:** *Summary of American Science Manpower, 1968,* Washington, D.C., 1970.

55 **Ward, P. D.:** *The History and Purposes of Regional Medical Programs,* unpublished paper, California Committee on Regional Medical Programs, San Francisco, 1967.

56 **U.S. Public Health Service:** *The Allied Health Professions Act of 1966 As Amended,* report to the President and the Congress, Washington, D.C., 1969.

Carnegie Commission on Higher Education
Publications in Print

HIGHER EDUCATION AND THE NATION'S HEALTH
a special report and recommendations by the Commission

GRADUATE AND PROFESSIONAL EDUCATION, 1980:
A SURVEY OF INSTITUTIONAL PLANS
Lewis B. Mayhew

THE AMERICAN COLLEGE AND AMERICAN CULTURE:
SOCIALIZATION AS A FUNCTION OF HIGHER EDUCATION
Oscar and Mary F. Handlin

RECENT ALUMNI AND HIGHER EDUCATION:
A SURVEY OF COLLEGE GRADUATES
Joe L. Spaeth and Andrew M. Greeley

CHANGE IN EDUCATIONAL POLICY:
SELF-STUDIES IN SELECTED COLLEGES AND UNIVERSITIES
Dwight R. Ladd

THE OPEN-DOOR COLLEGES:
POLICIES FOR COMMUNITY COLLEGES
a special report and recommendations by the Commission

QUALITY AND EQUALITY: REVISED RECOMMENDATIONS
NEW LEVELS OF FEDERAL RESPONSIBILITY FOR HIGHER EDUCATION
a supplement to the 1968 special report by the Commission

STATE OFFICIALS AND HIGHER EDUCATION:
A SURVEY OF THE OPINIONS AND EXPECTATIONS OF POLICY MAKERS IN NINE STATES
Heinz Eulau and Harold Quinley

A CHANCE TO LEARN:
AN ACTION AGENDA FOR EQUAL OPPORTUNITY IN HIGHER EDUCATION
a special report and recommendations by the Commission

ACADEMIC DEGREE STRUCTURES:
INNOVATIVE APPROACHES
PRINCIPLES OF REFORM IN DEGREE STRUCTURES IN THE UNITED STATES
Stephen H. Spurr

COLLEGES OF THE FORGOTTEN AMERICANS:
A PROFILE OF STATE COLLEGES AND REGIONAL UNIVERSITIES
E. Alden Dunham

FROM BACKWATER TO MAINSTREAM:
A PROFILE OF CATHOLIC HIGHER EDUCATION
Andrew M. Greeley

ALTERNATIVE METHODS OF FEDERAL FUNDING FOR HIGHER EDUCATION
Ron Wolk

INVENTORY OF CURRENT RESEARCH ON HIGHER EDUCATION 1968
Dale M. Heckman and Warren Bryan Martin

QUALITY AND EQUALITY:
NEW LEVELS OF FEDERAL RESPONSIBILITY FOR HIGHER EDUCATION
a special report and recommendations by the Commission, with 1970 revisions

The following reprints are available from the Carnegie Commission on Higher Education, 1947 Center Street, Berkeley, California 94704

RESOURCES FOR HIGHER EDUCATION:
AN ECONOMIST'S VIEW
Theodore W. Schultz

INDUSTRIAL RELATIONS AND UNIVERSITY
RELATIONS
Clark Kerr

STUDENT PROTEST — AN INSTITUTIONAL
AND NATIONAL PROFILE
Harold L. Hodgkinson

WHAT'S BUGGING THE STUDENTS?
Kenneth Keniston